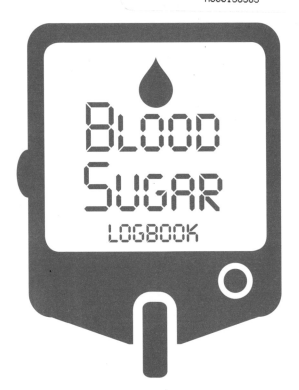

BLOOD SUGAR LOGBOOK

Daily Tracker for Optimum Wellness

Claudine Gandolfi

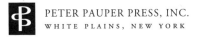

PETER PAUPER PRESS, INC.
WHITE PLAINS, NEW YORK

PETER PAUPER PRESS
Fine Books and Gifts Since 1928

Our Company

In 1928, at the age of twenty-two, Peter Beilenson began printing books on a small press in the basement of his parents' home in Larchmont, New York. Peter—and later, his wife, Edna—sought to create fine books that sold at "prices even a pauper could afford."

Today, still family owned and operated, Peter Pauper Press continues to honor our founders' legacy—and our customers' expectations—of beauty, quality, and value.

Designed by Tesslyn Pandarakalam
Images used under license from Shutterstock.com

Copyright © 2017
Peter Pauper Press, Inc.
202 Mamaroneck Avenue
White Plains, NY 10601
All rights reserved
ISBN 978-1-4413-2412-2
Printed in China
14 13 12 11 10 9 8

Visit us at www.peterpauper.com

This book is for general informational purposes only. It is not meant to substitute for the advice of a health care professional. Consult your physician before initiating any dietary or exercise program. Peter Pauper Press, Inc., makes no claims whatsoever regarding the use or interpretation of this book's content.

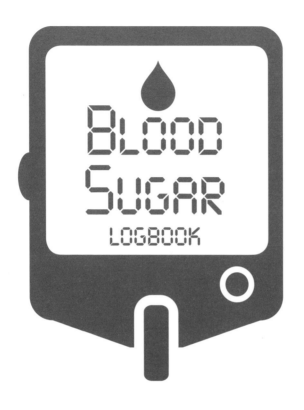

Daily Tracker for
Optimum Wellness

CONTENTS

INTRODUCTION

You're in charge of your own health and have wisely decided to keep track of your sugar intake. Some of you may be diabetic or pre-diabetic and trying to get your blood sugar under control. Others may simply know the pitfalls of sugar addiction and want to be healthier, lose weight, or feel better. And some are using a diet plan to break the sugar cycle's highs and lows.

The most important thing to do before you start is to consult with your doctor to see what is right for you. If you're on medications, that will need to be taken into account. Consider what your specific goals are and work with your doctor, dietician, or endocrinologist to come up with a plan that best fits your needs.

Whether you're following a doctor's prescribed plan, or you just need a place to log your current health goals, we've got you covered. Are you doing the latest belly fat or blood sugar or glycemic index and beyond diet? Whatever your personal preference, this logbook can be customized to meet your specific needs and goals. There's room in the log pages to record what you're eating so that you can keep an eye on your general health and weight. And if you're planning on exercising, which is recommended, you can keep track of that in the log pages as well.

USING THE BLOOD SUGAR LOGBOOK

How to Fill Out the Daily Blood Sugar Log Pages

This book has been created for you to record what you're eating. It should last you about three and a half months. In the Daily Blood Sugar Log section beginning on page 19, you'll write in the day, date, and the week number that you're currently recording on the top left of each page. The log pages are designed to be adaptable to whether you use the log daily or not. See the sample Daily Blood Sugar Log entry on the right for reference.

You should fill out the log as completely as possible. If you're on insulin and keeping track of your pre- and post-meal blood sugar levels, as well as the dose of insulin you're using, fill in those figures in the blue row next to each meal.

The majority of the logbook is for you to record what you've eaten each day. You'll keep track of your carbs, as well as other nutrients in your food. We've also included columns to keep track of the glycemic load of your meals. This can be helpful in keeping your blood sugar even throughout the day. The Nutritional Facts section in the back includes glycemic index and glycemic load figures for many common foods. We've included a column for "other" nutrients you may want to track—like points if you're on Weight Watchers® or salt if you're monitoring that.

There's space at the top of the pages to rate your mood and energy levels. At the bottom of the pages, there's a place to record your vitamins/supplements, activity or exercise, and notes.

As you go back and review these pages once complete, you should be able to notice trends. If you eat too many carbs, how does that affect your energy level? What if you eat too little? You can moderate your intake of various nutrients to determine where you're most comfortable, healthy, and energetic.

DAILY BLOOD SUGAR LOG

DAY/DATE: _Thursday 5 / 8 / 20_

WEIGHT: _210_

MOOD/ENERGY: _Good/average_

	Glycemic index	Glycemic load	Calories (kcal)	Carbs (g)	Fiber (g)	Total sugar (g)	Added sugar (g)	Protein (g)
BREAKFAST / TIME: 7:30 INSULIN:			PRE SUGAR LEVEL:			POST SUGAR LEVEL:		
blueberry muffin (2.1 oz)	50±3	15	180	31	1	22	18	2
egg whites (1/2 cup)	----	----	60	0	0	0	0	6
BREAKFAST TOTALS		15	240	31	1	22	18	8
SNACK / TIME: 10:00								
yogurt (plain, lowfat) (7.1 oz)	33±7	10	154	17	0	17	0	13
LUNCH / TIME: 1:30 INSULIN:			PRE SUGAR LEVEL:			POST SUGAR LEVEL:		
grilled chicken (4 oz)	----	----	142	0	0	0	0	27
grape tomatoes (3 oz)	----	----	14	3	1	0	0	1
romaine (2 cups)	----	----	20	3	1	0	0	1
pita bread (1.1 oz)	68±5	10	82	17	1	0	0	3
LUNCH TOTALS		10	258	23	3	0	0	32
SNACK / TIME: 3:30								
apple (1 small)	39±3	6	62	17	3	11	0	0
DINNER / TIME: 7:00 INSULIN:			PRE SUGAR LEVEL:			POST SUGAR LEVEL:		
skirt steak (4 oz)	----	----	200	0	0	0	0	21
sweet potato (5.3 oz)	70±6	22	129	30	5	6	0	2
broccoli (1 cup)	----	----	30	6	2	2	0	3
DINNER TOTALS		22	359	36	7	8	0	26
SNACK / TIME: 8:30								
roasted cashews (1.8 oz)	25±1	3	287	16	2	1	0	8
DAILY TOTALS:		66	1,360	140	16	59	18	87

VITAMINS / SUPPLEMENTS: _Multi, vit C (500), essential fatty acids_

EXERCISE: _2-mile walk, free weights (upper body)_

NOTES: _Felt tired until afternoon walk—then energized!_

KEEPING TRACK OF CARBS

Your body uses carbohydrates for energy. Made of simpler molecules than protein or fat, carbohydrates are the nutrient most easily used by your body. This is why marathon runners often carb-load before a race. The body will be able to run on that accessible fuel for a longer period of time. Because it's the easiest for the body to break down, it's also the one that gets stored fastest. Carbs are digested and converted to glucose in the blood. If you burn up that fuel, all is well. If you don't, then it gets stored as glycogen in the liver and muscles. When the body needs a reserve of energy it converts the glycogen back into glucose for fuel. So, why are you reading all of this simple science? Because when your body uses carbs and stores carbs, it's not going to use the fat and protein you're eating, since they take longer to break down. Protein is actually used as a last resort for fuel by the body simply because there are so many other places the protein needs to be used (such as building and repairing muscle, and delivering oxygen). The more excess carbs you consume, the more everything will be stored. This translates into weight gain.

If you've ever tried to exercise while on a low carb/high protein diet, you've probably felt energy drain much quicker than while you were on a balanced diet. That's because your body burns carbs and their glucose first, then it will re-convert the glycogen in the liver and muscles back to glucose, and then the fat stored there, too. So, if you're eating high protein, that will be the last thing your body will try to use as fuel. With very few carbs to draw on, the body must use its energy to convert glycogen back to glucose or metabolize the fat stores. Still with me?

What Kind of Carbs Are Bad?

The simple carbs (you know the drill—white flour, white sugar, potatoes, pasta, and white rice) are the easiest ones for the body to break down, absorbing quickly into the bloodstream and causing a rapid rise in blood sugar. If you can avoid these, it's probably for the best. Think back to before the industrial revolution. How easy were sweets and cereals to come by? They weren't. Mankind invented this particular monkey on our back by refining sugar cane, and our health has suffered since. Refined sugar has almost drug-like addictive tendencies and poisonous effects when heavily consumed. But does that mean all carbs are bad? Far from it.

What Kind of Carbs Are Best?

Since carbohydrates are your body's preferred and easiest form of fuel, you just have to make sure you're not eating too many. Your body needs some, so it's not a good idea—and probably not even possible—to completely cut out all carbs. Try to focus on the "slow burn" food items with complex carbs. Those are the ones that take your body longer to process because they have fiber or some protein in them: whole grain breads and pastas, legumes, brown rice, fruits and vegetables. Yes, that's right. Fruits and veggies contain mostly carbs, but they're very good for you because they're not just simple carbs. Complex carbs won't spike your blood sugar like simple carbs do.

Vitamins/Supplements

If you're taking any vitamins or supplements, this book is the perfect place to keep track of them. Make sure to indicate the strength (1000 IU, 100 mg, etc.) as well as dosage, so you can determine how much works best for your body. You can also list your other medications in this section.

Exercise

If you are tracking blood sugar, you might notice your levels are higher after exercising. Once your body has used the few minutes of carbs in your digestive system, it's going to call for the reserves (glycogen) stored in your cells to be released. That will raise your blood sugar. Don't be alarmed. If you're diabetic, keep in mind that the excess glucose released in your blood due to exercise will need insulin in order to be used by your muscles. Consult your doctor about any exercise program you undertake. Always carry a carb snack with you.

If you're not a diabetic, you should still consult with a doctor before you begin an exercise regimen. You'll find a combination of cardio, strength training, and flexibility exercises optimal for health and vitality.

Notes

Feel free to record anything you like on this line at the bottom of each daily log page. Maybe the weather is affecting you? Bad day at work? It's sometimes easier to see trends and connections when you have it down on paper, and that can help you make course corrections.

Sugar – The Bad and the Ugly

Historically, sugar was an expensive sweetener that not all could afford, and as such, was used sparingly. Only in the last 200 years or so has sugar been mass-produced and affordable. It has become increasingly clear that sugar contributes to a wide variety of health problems. To make matters worse, the last 40 years have seen the introduction of another unhealthy sweetener into the mainstream diet: high-fructose corn syrup (HFCS). It's inexpensive, easy to produce, and a boon to the corn industry.

Sugar is a lucrative business, and those who profit from it have significant incentive to deny its health risks. The possible link between sugar and heart disease has only lately become public knowledge. We have also acquired a greater understanding of sugar and addiction—studies demonstrate that eating it makes you crave more.

The World Health Organization Dietary Guidelines in 2015 recommended that added sugars comprise less than ten percent of one's total daily calories, and that further limiting free sugar to less than five percent of daily calories would provide additional health benefits. The American Heart Association recommends no more than 150 calories or 9 teaspoons of sugar per day for men, and 100 calories or 6 teaspoons of sugar per day for women. (There are 16 calories in a teaspoon of sugar.) For perspective, there are more than 8 teaspoons (33 grams) of sugar in a 12-ounce can of soda. Americans consume an average of 19.5 teaspoons daily.

Effective July 2018, the U.S. Food and Drug Administration (FDA) is requiring a more sugar-conscious Nutrition Facts label on packaged foods. It turns out that added sugars were never listed under sugars on those labels but lumped in under Carbohydrates. The new updated label includes added sugars under sugars, as well as broken out separately.

U.S. Food & Drug Administration, *Highlights of What's Different on the New Label*

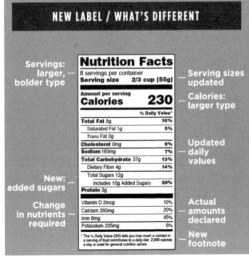

10

DIABETES AND BLOOD SUGAR

While this logbook can serve many purposes, helping to track blood sugar if you're a diabetic is one of them. Proper nutrition can help bring your blood sugar spikes under control. The trick to maintaining a healthy blood sugar level is consistency. Peaks and valleys are pitfalls you want to avoid so you can lessen and—if you're Type II—possibly even cease taking insulin. Unfortunately, you may have noticed that you gained weight once you started taking insulin. This is common. This logbook can help you get that under control and regain your health.

In Type I diabetes, the pancreas simply has stopped producing insulin and there is no getting around that with your diet. In Type II, you produce insulin but your body has grown immune to its effects. This logbook can be a useful tool in keeping track of how many carbs you've consumed and where your levels are at any given time, helping you identify and address trends.

Testing Your Blood Sugar Levels

You can use your meter to record and keep track of your blood sugar levels before and after meals. The logbook provides areas for this on the far right of each Daily Blood Sugar Log page. There's also an area for you to record the amount of medication you are currently taking.

Consult with your health practitioner for your own ideal range of blood sugar levels. There will be an increase in blood sugar after you've eaten, but after a few hours it will return back to normal. It's when the body can't get back to where it should be that the problem arises.

Controlling Blood Sugar Through Diet

Some things will be obvious—avoid sugary, processed snacks, or skip the frappaccinos and just have a cup of regular coffee. Eat natural, unprocessed foods as much as possible (As fitness guru Jack LaLanne said, "If man made it, don't eat it."), and avoid sweetened drinks and juices. Seek out low carb, low sugar vegetables and fruits.

DIETS THAT FOCUS ON BLOOD SUGAR

There are several diet plans that cater to blood sugar concerns, so perhaps you can find one that works for you to help control your weight, manage your mood swings, keep your diabetes in check, or simply get healthy. There's obviously a reason why these diets are prevalent today. Sugar is addictive, and simple sugar is a relatively modern concoction that has destructive tendencies in our blood. Below is a list of some of the more popular diets for your information only. Please note that many of these diets claim to help you lose weight and manage your health, but not all diets are healthy for everyone. Use this list as a starting point for your own research before deciding to commit to a diet.

More importantly, consult your doctor before beginning any new diet, especially if you have health issues or a history of disordered eating.

Glycemic Index

Premise: Developed by the University of Sydney and followed globally, the Glycemic Index (GI) is a guide that breaks down foods that contain carbs into categories that can help you track which are better for keeping your blood sugar constant. Foods with a high GI will quickly spike your blood sugar, so those with an index of 55 or below (low GI) are optimal for keeping yourself "in tune," minimizing cravings and propensities to binge. Keeping insulin levels balanced helps you feel full, and you may be less likely to snack between meals because your energy level is already up. The Glycemic Load (GL) is the grams of carbs in a food times the food's GI, divided by 100. The higher the number, the worse for your blood sugar it is. We've included the GI here in the logbook just to make it clear which fruits and vegetables are easier for your body to handle while maintaining a constant blood sugar level. A lot of other diets have taken the low GI approach to nutrition, and built upon what the University of Sydney developed.

The Paleo Diet

Premise: Dr. Loren Cordain wants you to eat like a caveman! This popular diet applies the principle of eating only what our forebears would have had available to them: no wheat, dairy, grains, beans, or sugar. This is a low glycemic load, high protein diet with an abundance of Omega 3 fats. It is recommended that you take vitamin D3 and fish oil supplements. There is an 85/15 rule that comes into play on this diet. You can have 3 meals a week that fall outside of the plan.

Blood Sugar Solution

Premise: Through a series of quizzes, Dr. Mark Hyman helps you self-diagnose for possible "diabesity," a word he coined that means the growing epidemic of diabetes and obesity, which he claims are linked. Most people, he claims, are pre-diabetic diabese and are deficient in important nutrients like Omega-3, magnesium, vitamin D, etc. He argues that inflammation, thyroid issues, depression, and more are caused by nutritional issues with dairy, sugar, flour, artificial sweeteners, food sensitivities, and more. Through an elimination diet and following his regimen of eating nothing from a package, nothing with added sugars, nothing with more than five ingredients, nothing hydrogenated, and nothing with caffeine or alcohol, he says that people can achieve ideal blood sugar, weight, and health goals.

Eat-Clean Diet®

Premise: Eat nothing packaged, nothing artificial. Sweeten, Tosca Reno says, only if you must, with natural sweeteners like agave and honey. Eat five to six small meals a day, starting with breakfast within thirty minutes of waking, and watch portion size but don't count calories. Make sure you're getting a complex carb and lean protein at each meal and that you're drinking eight to twelve cups of water a day. This plan aims to increase your vitality and energy exponentially.

Master Your Metabolism

Premise: Eat nothing with refined sugars or processed grains, and eat many small meals a day—but nothing after 9 PM. Avoid soy, and make sure to get in your ten "power nutrient" foods: legumes, alliums, berries, meat and eggs, colorful fruit and veggies, cruciferous veggies, dark green leafy veggies, nuts and seeds, organic low-fat dairy, and whole grains. Avoid anything artificial and get in plenty of exercise. Don't make Jillian Michaels come whip your behind!

Every Other Day Diet/Fast Diet®

Premise: Every other day (or two out of five days, depending on which you choose), you fast, eating no more than 500 calories if you're a woman, or 600 if you're a man. According to many studies, intermittent fasting and avoidance of white sugars and carbs with high GI can help you live longer and be healthier. While no study suggests such a diet would put your body into starvation mode or lower your metabolism, it's also important to note that there is inconsistent evidence concerning whether or not intermittent fasting is safe for all dieters.

TRACKING CALORIES—LOSING WEIGHT & BUILDING MUSCLE

If you're trying to lose weight and/or build muscle, calories play a huge factor. If you learn to track your calories and pay attention to not only the amount of calories, but the types of calories (i.e. protein vs. carbs), you'll be way ahead of the game.

Basal Metabolic Rate

Welcome to your Basal Metabolic Rate! Your BMR indicates the calories your body needs per day to survive without moving. If you're awake and sitting, but not exercising, multiply that number by 1.2—the result is the amount of calories you need to maintain weight. You can also estimate this figure by using the calorie calculator at www.mayoclinic.com. Trying to lose weight? You'll need to cut calories and increase exercise in order to maintain muscle mass. If you don't ingest enough calories for the day, you'll do more harm than good. In general, if you're trying to lose weight, it's recommended to aim for a loss of 1 to 2 pounds a week, no more.

Here's the formula:

Women: BMR = 655 + (4.35 x weight in lbs) + (4.7 x height in inches) – (4.7 x age in years)

or metric: 655.1 + (9.56 x weight in kg) + (1.85 x height in cm) – (4.68 x age in years)

Men: BMR = 66 + (6.23 x weight in lbs) + (12.7 x height in inches) – (6.8 x age in years)

or metric: 66.5 + (13.75 x weight in kg) + (5 x height in cm) – (6.76 x age in years)

Daily Recommended Caloric Intake

If you're following a traditional diet, you'll be counting calories. Once you have calculated your BMR, you can then figure out how many calories you should be aiming for daily if you're trying to lose weight. If you reduce net calories (by eating 500 fewer calories a day and/or exercising), you'll be able to lose 1 pound a week. You need 3,500 fewer calories than required by your BMR to burn off a pound (500 x 7 days = 3,500 calories). However, keep in mind that even if you're trying to lose weight, many sources recommend that calories consumed should be no less than 1,200 for women and 1,800 for men.

> **Note:** Consuming too few calories will not necessarily get you to your goal faster. In the past, it was believed that cutting calories from your diet will force your body to consume its own muscle mass to compensate for its lack of energy stores, but recent studies have shown this is only the case after months of calorie deprivation. However, as noted in the previous section on dieting, studies have also shown that depriving your body of calories puts stress on your body and may lead to other adverse side-effects. Always consult your doctor before cutting anything from your diet, and never starve yourself!

For those who are normal weight but trying to bulk up and build muscle mass, it's suggested to add about 250–500 calories to your diet per day. Try adding some lean protein to your daily intake. It's best to eat this about twenty minutes before and up to an hour after your strength training for optimal effect. To gain muscle you should be consuming about 1 to 1.5 times your body weight in grams of lean protein a day.

What are some examples of a "lean" protein?
- Eggs
- Whey or soy protein (supplements available as powder or bars)
- Grilled or baked chicken/turkey breast
- Non-fat Greek yogurt
- Salmon and other fish
- Bean, legumes, and whole grains

Body Mass Index

The dreaded Body Mass Index! A good indicator of body fatness, your BMI should stay below 25. The formula below tells you how to find yours. Height is measured without shoes and weight without clothes.

$$\text{BMI} = 703 \quad \text{x} \quad \frac{\text{weight in lbs}}{\text{height in inches}^2} \qquad \text{or} \qquad \frac{\text{weight in kg}}{\text{height in m}^2}$$

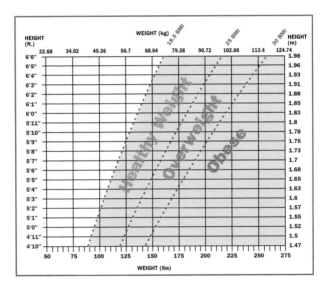

Here are guidelines for healthy body fat percentages, by age and gender. You can ascertain your body fat with a specialized scale or with help from a personal trainer.*

AGE	WOMEN	MEN
20-39	21% to 32%	8% to 19%
40-59	23% to 33%	11% to 21%
60 and up	24% to 35%	13% to 24%

*In addition, BMI should be between 18.5 and 24.9

TRACKING YOUR PROGRESS

Depending on what your specific goals are, you may choose to track your progress in different ways. The lower your resting heart rate, the better your cardiovascular health, so you may want to keep track of that. Or you may be interested in recalculating your BMR as it changes due to any variances in your weight. Some people like to use their Body Mass Index (BMI) as a tool to track their progress. (*See more info about calculating your BMI on previous pages.*) In addition to, or instead of, tracking your weight, you may take weekly measurements of your arms, legs, waist, etc. You can record any of this information in the Observations/Notes section at the bottom left of the log pages.

When you first begin exercising, you may drop a nice chunk of weight almost immediately. I like to think of this as a gift. Yes, it's mostly water weight, but it sure is encouraging! Just don't give up if you don't see the same results in the second and third week. By that time, you're actually burning fat stores—that takes longer to lose than water. Whether it's weight, measurements, or anything else you're tracking, use this logbook as a positive, motivating tool. Go you!

*To ensure good health: eat lightly,
breathe deeply, live moderately,
cultivate cheerfulness,
and maintain
an interest in life.*

—WILLIAM LONDEN

HELPFUL ONLINE RESOURCES

NUTRITION INFORMATION

www.usda.gov

www.diabetes.org

www.dietaryguidelines.gov

www.caloriecontrol.org

www.choosemyplate.gov

www.webmd.com

www.nutritiondata.com

www.cspinet.org/nah

www.hsph.harvard.edu/nutritionsource

www.nhlbi.nih.gov/health/public/heart/
obesity/lose_wt/index.htm

www.realage.com

www.myfooddiary.com

www.livestrong.com/thedailyplate

www.food.gov.uk

www.nutrition.org.uk

www.dh.gov.uk/en/Publichealth/Nutrition/
index.htm

BLOOD SUGAR DIETS

www.glycemicindex.com

www.bloodsugarsolution.com

www.jillianmichaels.com

www.thepaleodiet.com/

FITNESS TECHNIQUES

www.fitnessonline.com

www.fitnessmagazine.com

www.fitness.gov

www.muscleandfitness.com

www.acsm.org

www.nsca-lift.org

www.acefitness.org

www.nasm.org

www.prohealth.com/weightloss

www.nhs.uk/livewell/fitness

SUPPORT

http://win.niddk.nih.gov/publications/
better_health.htm

www.weightwatchers.com

www.jennycraig.com

www.ediets.com

http://dwlz.com

www.hungry-girl.com

DAILY
BLOOD SUGAR
Log Pages

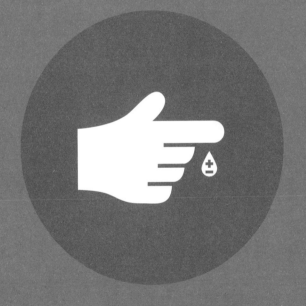

We are what we repeatedly do.
Excellence, then, is not an act, but a habit.
—ARISTOTLE

DAILY BLOOD SUGAR LOG

DAY/DATE: _____

WEIGHT: _____

MOOD/ENERGY: _____

	Glycemic index	Glycemic load	Calories (kcal)	Carbs (g)	Fiber (g)	Total sugar (g)	Added sugar (g)	Protein (g)
BREAKFAST / TIME:	INSULIN:		PRE SUGAR LEVEL:			POST SUGAR LEVEL:		
BREAKFAST TOTALS								
SNACK / TIME:								
LUNCH / TIME:	INSULIN:		PRE SUGAR LEVEL:			POST SUGAR LEVEL:		
LUNCH TOTALS								
SNACK / TIME:								
DINNER / TIME:	INSULIN:		PRE SUGAR LEVEL:			POST SUGAR LEVEL:		
DINNER TOTALS								
SNACK / TIME:								
DAILY TOTALS:								

VITAMINS / SUPPLEMENTS:

EXERCISE:

NOTES:

DAILY BLOOD SUGAR LOG

DAY/DATE: _____

WEIGHT: _____

MOOD/ENERGY: _____

	Glycemic index	Glycemic load	Calories (kcal)	Carbs (g)	Fiber (g)	Total sugar (g)	Added sugar (g)	Protein (g)
BREAKFAST / TIME: **INSULIN:** **PRE SUGAR LEVEL:** **POST SUGAR LEVEL:**								
BREAKFAST TOTALS								
SNACK / TIME:								
LUNCH / TIME: **INSULIN:** **PRE SUGAR LEVEL:** **POST SUGAR LEVEL:**								
LUNCH TOTALS								
SNACK / TIME:								
DINNER / TIME: **INSULIN:** **PRE SUGAR LEVEL:** **POST SUGAR LEVEL:**								
DINNER TOTALS								
SNACK / TIME:								
DAILY TOTALS:								

VITAMINS / SUPPLEMENTS:

EXERCISE:

NOTES:

DAILY BLOOD SUGAR LOG

DAY / DATE: _____

WEIGHT: _____

MOOD / ENERGY: _____

	Glycemic index	Glycemic load	Calories (kcal)	Carbs (g)	Fiber (g)	Total sugar (g)	Added sugar (g)	Protein (g)
BREAKFAST / TIME: **INSULIN:** **PRE SUGAR LEVEL:** **POST SUGAR LEVEL:**								
BREAKFAST TOTALS								
SNACK / TIME:								
LUNCH / TIME: **INSULIN:** **PRE SUGAR LEVEL:** **POST SUGAR LEVEL:**								
LUNCH TOTALS								
SNACK / TIME:								
DINNER / TIME: **INSULIN:** **PRE SUGAR LEVEL:** **POST SUGAR LEVEL:**								
DINNER TOTALS								
SNACK / TIME:								
DAILY TOTALS:								

VITAMINS / SUPPLEMENTS:
_____

EXERCISE:
_____

NOTES:
_____

DAILY BLOOD SUGAR LOG

DAY/DATE: _____

WEIGHT: _____

MOOD/ENERGY: _____

	Glycemic index	Glycemic load	Calories (kcal)	Carbs (g)	Fiber (g)	Total sugar (g)	Added sugar (g)	Protein (g)
BREAKFAST / TIME: INSULIN: PRE SUGAR LEVEL: POST SUGAR LEVEL:								
BREAKFAST TOTALS								
SNACK / TIME:								
LUNCH / TIME: INSULIN: PRE SUGAR LEVEL: POST SUGAR LEVEL:								
LUNCH TOTALS								
SNACK / TIME:								
DINNER / TIME: INSULIN: PRE SUGAR LEVEL: POST SUGAR LEVEL:								
DINNER TOTALS								
SNACK / TIME:								
DAILY TOTALS:								

VITAMINS / SUPPLEMENTS:

EXERCISE:

NOTES:

DAILY BLOOD SUGAR LOG

DAY/DATE: _____

WEIGHT: _____

MOOD/ENERGY: _____

	Glycemic index	Glycemic load	Calories (kcal)	Carbs (g)	Fiber (g)	Total sugar (g)	Added sugar (g)	Protein (g)
BREAKFAST / TIME: **INSULIN:** **PRE SUGAR LEVEL:** **POST SUGAR LEVEL:**								
BREAKFAST TOTALS								
SNACK / TIME:								
LUNCH / TIME: **INSULIN:** **PRE SUGAR LEVEL:** **POST SUGAR LEVEL:**								
LUNCH TOTALS								
SNACK / TIME:								
DINNER / TIME: **INSULIN:** **PRE SUGAR LEVEL:** **POST SUGAR LEVEL:**								
DINNER TOTALS								
SNACK / TIME:								
DAILY TOTALS:								

VITAMINS / SUPPLEMENTS:

EXERCISE:

NOTES:

DAILY BLOOD SUGAR LOG

DAY/DATE: _____

WEIGHT: _____

MOOD/ENERGY: _____

	Glycemic index	Glycemic load	Calories (kcal)	Carbs (g)	Fiber (g)	Total sugar (g)	Added sugar (g)	Protein (g)
BREAKFAST / TIME: INSULIN: PRE SUGAR LEVEL: POST SUGAR LEVEL:								
BREAKFAST TOTALS								
SNACK / TIME:								
LUNCH / TIME: INSULIN: PRE SUGAR LEVEL: POST SUGAR LEVEL:								
LUNCH TOTALS								
SNACK / TIME:								
DINNER / TIME: INSULIN: PRE SUGAR LEVEL: POST SUGAR LEVEL:								
DINNER TOTALS								
SNACK / TIME:								
DAILY TOTALS:								

VITAMINS / SUPPLEMENTS: _____

EXERCISE: _____

NOTES: _____

DAILY BLOOD SUGAR LOG

DAY/DATE: _____

WEIGHT: _____

MOOD/ENERGY: _____

	Glycemic index	Glycemic load	Calories (kcal)	Carbs (g)	Fiber (g)	Total sugar (g)	Added sugar (g)	Protein (g)
BREAKFAST / TIME: ___ **INSULIN:** ___ **PRE SUGAR LEVEL:** ___ **POST SUGAR LEVEL:** ___								
BREAKFAST TOTALS								
SNACK / TIME: ___								
LUNCH / TIME: ___ **INSULIN:** ___ **PRE SUGAR LEVEL:** ___ **POST SUGAR LEVEL:** ___								
LUNCH TOTALS								
SNACK / TIME: ___								
DINNER / TIME: ___ **INSULIN:** ___ **PRE SUGAR LEVEL:** ___ **POST SUGAR LEVEL:** ___								
DINNER TOTALS								
SNACK / TIME: ___								
DAILY TOTALS:								

VITAMINS / SUPPLEMENTS:
_____

EXERCISE:
_____
_____

NOTES:
_____

DAILY BLOOD SUGAR LOG

DAY/DATE: _____

WEIGHT: _____

MOOD/ENERGY: _____

	Glycemic index	Glycemic load	Calories (kcal)	Carbs (g)	Fiber (g)	Total sugar (g)	Added sugar (g)	Protein (g)
BREAKFAST / TIME: ___ **INSULIN:** ___ **PRE SUGAR LEVEL:** ___ **POST SUGAR LEVEL:** ___								
BREAKFAST TOTALS								
SNACK / TIME: ___								
LUNCH / TIME: ___ **INSULIN:** ___ **PRE SUGAR LEVEL:** ___ **POST SUGAR LEVEL:** ___								
LUNCH TOTALS								
SNACK / TIME: ___								
DINNER / TIME: ___ **INSULIN:** ___ **PRE SUGAR LEVEL:** ___ **POST SUGAR LEVEL:** ___								
DINNER TOTALS								
SNACK / TIME: ___								
DAILY TOTALS:								

VITAMINS / SUPPLEMENTS: _____

EXERCISE: _____

NOTES: _____

DAILY BLOOD SUGAR LOG

DAY/DATE: _____

WEIGHT: _____

MOOD/ENERGY: _____

	Glycemic index	Glycemic load	Calories (kcal)	Carbs (g)	Fiber (g)	Total sugar (g)	Added sugar (g)	Protein (g)
BREAKFAST / TIME:	INSULIN:		PRE SUGAR LEVEL:			POST SUGAR LEVEL:		
BREAKFAST TOTALS								
SNACK / TIME:								
LUNCH / TIME:	INSULIN:		PRE SUGAR LEVEL:			POST SUGAR LEVEL:		
LUNCH TOTALS								
SNACK / TIME:								
DINNER / TIME:	INSULIN:		PRE SUGAR LEVEL:			POST SUGAR LEVEL:		
DINNER TOTALS								
SNACK / TIME:								
DAILY TOTALS:								

VITAMINS / SUPPLEMENTS: _____

EXERCISE: _____

NOTES: _____

DAILY BLOOD SUGAR LOG

DAY / DATE: _____

WEIGHT: _____

MOOD / ENERGY: _____

	Glycemic index	Glycemic load	Calories (kcal)	Carbs (g)	Fiber (g)	Total sugar (g)	Added sugar (g)	Protein (g)
BREAKFAST / TIME: _____ **INSULIN:** _____ **PRE SUGAR LEVEL:** _____ **POST SUGAR LEVEL:** _____								
BREAKFAST TOTALS								
SNACK / TIME: _____								
LUNCH / TIME: _____ **INSULIN:** _____ **PRE SUGAR LEVEL:** _____ **POST SUGAR LEVEL:** _____								
LUNCH TOTALS								
SNACK / TIME: _____								
DINNER / TIME: _____ **INSULIN:** _____ **PRE SUGAR LEVEL:** _____ **POST SUGAR LEVEL:** _____								
DINNER TOTALS								
SNACK / TIME: _____								
DAILY TOTALS:								

VITAMINS / SUPPLEMENTS:

_____

_____

EXERCISE:

_____

_____

NOTES:

_____

DAILY BLOOD SUGAR LOG

DAY/DATE: _____

WEIGHT: _____

MOOD/ENERGY: _____

	Glycemic index	Glycemic load	Calories (Kcal)	Carbs (g)	Fiber (g)	Total sugar (g)	Added sugar (g)	Protein (g)
BREAKFAST / TIME: ___ **INSULIN:** ___ **PRE SUGAR LEVEL:** ___ **POST SUGAR LEVEL:** ___								
BREAKFAST TOTALS								
SNACK / TIME: ___								
LUNCH / TIME: ___ **INSULIN:** ___ **PRE SUGAR LEVEL:** ___ **POST SUGAR LEVEL:** ___								
LUNCH TOTALS								
SNACK / TIME: ___								
DINNER / TIME: ___ **INSULIN:** ___ **PRE SUGAR LEVEL:** ___ **POST SUGAR LEVEL:** ___								
DINNER TOTALS								
SNACK / TIME: ___								
DAILY TOTALS:								

VITAMINS / SUPPLEMENTS:
_____

EXERCISE:
_____

NOTES:
_____

DAILY BLOOD SUGAR LOG

DAY/DATE: _____

WEIGHT: _____

MOOD/ENERGY: _____

	Glycemic index	Glycemic load	Calories (kcal)	Carbs (g)	Fiber (g)	Total sugar (g)	Added sugar (g)	Protein (g)
BREAKFAST / TIME: _____ **INSULIN:** _____ **PRE SUGAR LEVEL:** _____ **POST SUGAR LEVEL:** _____								
BREAKFAST TOTALS								
SNACK / TIME: _____								
LUNCH / TIME: _____ **INSULIN:** _____ **PRE SUGAR LEVEL:** _____ **POST SUGAR LEVEL:** _____								
LUNCH TOTALS								
SNACK / TIME: _____								
DINNER / TIME: _____ **INSULIN:** _____ **PRE SUGAR LEVEL:** _____ **POST SUGAR LEVEL:** _____								
DINNER TOTALS								
SNACK / TIME: _____								
DAILY TOTALS:								

VITAMINS / SUPPLEMENTS:

EXERCISE:

NOTES:

DAILY BLOOD SUGAR LOG

DAY/DATE: _____

WEIGHT: _____

MOOD/ENERGY: _____

	Glycemic index	Glycemic load	Calories (kcal)	Carbs (g)	Fiber (g)	Total sugar (g)	Added sugar (g)	Protein (g)
BREAKFAST / TIME: INSULIN: PRE SUGAR LEVEL: POST SUGAR LEVEL:								
BREAKFAST TOTALS								
SNACK / TIME:								
LUNCH / TIME: INSULIN: PRE SUGAR LEVEL: POST SUGAR LEVEL:								
LUNCH TOTALS								
SNACK / TIME:								
DINNER / TIME: INSULIN: PRE SUGAR LEVEL: POST SUGAR LEVEL:								
DINNER TOTALS								
SNACK / TIME:								
DAILY TOTALS:								

VITAMINS / SUPPLEMENTS:

EXERCISE:

NOTES:

DAILY BLOOD SUGAR LOG

DAY/DATE: _____

WEIGHT: _____

MOOD/ENERGY: _____

	Glycemic index	Glycemic load	Calories (kcal)	Carbs (g)	Fiber (g)	Total sugar (g)	Added sugar (g)	Protein (g)
BREAKFAST / TIME: **INSULIN:** **PRE SUGAR LEVEL:** **POST SUGAR LEVEL:**								
BREAKFAST TOTALS								
SNACK / TIME:								
LUNCH / TIME: **INSULIN:** **PRE SUGAR LEVEL:** **POST SUGAR LEVEL:**								
LUNCH TOTALS								
SNACK / TIME:								
DINNER / TIME: **INSULIN:** **PRE SUGAR LEVEL:** **POST SUGAR LEVEL:**								
DINNER TOTALS								
SNACK / TIME:								
DAILY TOTALS:								

VITAMINS / SUPPLEMENTS:

EXERCISE:

NOTES:

DAILY BLOOD SUGAR LOG

DAY/DATE: _____

WEIGHT: _____

MOOD/ENERGY: _____

	Glycemic index	Glycemic load	Calories (kcal)	Carbs (g)	Fiber (g)	Total sugar (g)	Added sugar (g)	Protein (g)
BREAKFAST / TIME: ☐ **INSULIN:** ☐ **PRE SUGAR LEVEL:** ☐ **POST SUGAR LEVEL:** ☐								
BREAKFAST TOTALS								
SNACK / TIME: ☐								
LUNCH / TIME: ☐ **INSULIN:** ☐ **PRE SUGAR LEVEL:** ☐ **POST SUGAR LEVEL:** ☐								
LUNCH TOTALS								
SNACK / TIME: ☐								
DINNER / TIME: ☐ **INSULIN:** ☐ **PRE SUGAR LEVEL:** ☐ **POST SUGAR LEVEL:** ☐								
DINNER TOTALS								
SNACK / TIME: ☐								
DAILY TOTALS:								

VITAMINS / SUPPLEMENTS:

EXERCISE:

NOTES:

DAILY BLOOD SUGAR LOG

DAY / DATE: _____

WEIGHT: _____

MOOD / ENERGY: _____

	Glycemic index	Glycemic load	Calories (kcal)	Carbs (g)	Fiber (g)	Total sugar (g)	Added sugar (g)	Protein (g)
BREAKFAST / TIME: **INSULIN:** **PRE SUGAR LEVEL:** **POST SUGAR LEVEL:**								
BREAKFAST TOTALS								
SNACK / TIME:								
LUNCH / TIME: **INSULIN:** **PRE SUGAR LEVEL:** **POST SUGAR LEVEL:**								
LUNCH TOTALS								
SNACK / TIME:								
DINNER / TIME: **INSULIN:** **PRE SUGAR LEVEL:** **POST SUGAR LEVEL:**								
DINNER TOTALS								
SNACK / TIME:								
DAILY TOTALS:								

VITAMINS / SUPPLEMENTS:

_____

EXERCISE:

_____

NOTES:

_____

DAILY BLOOD SUGAR LOG

DAY/DATE: _____

WEIGHT: _____

MOOD/ENERGY: _____

	Glycemic index	Glycemic load	Calories (kcal)	Carbs (g)	Fiber (g)	Total sugar (g)	Added sugar (g)	Protein (g)
BREAKFAST / TIME: **INSULIN:** **PRE SUGAR LEVEL:** **POST SUGAR LEVEL:**								
BREAKFAST TOTALS								
SNACK / TIME:								
LUNCH / TIME: **INSULIN:** **PRE SUGAR LEVEL:** **POST SUGAR LEVEL:**								
LUNCH TOTALS								
SNACK / TIME:								
DINNER / TIME: **INSULIN:** **PRE SUGAR LEVEL:** **POST SUGAR LEVEL:**								
DINNER TOTALS								
SNACK / TIME:								
DAILY TOTALS:								

VITAMINS / SUPPLEMENTS:

EXERCISE:

NOTES:

DAILY BLOOD SUGAR LOG

DAY/DATE: _____

WEIGHT: _____

MOOD/ENERGY: _____

	Glycemic index	Glycemic load	Calories (kcal)	Carbs (g)	Fiber (g)	Total sugar (g)	Added sugar (g)	Protein (g)
BREAKFAST / TIME: **INSULIN:** **PRE SUGAR LEVEL:** **POST SUGAR LEVEL:**								
BREAKFAST TOTALS								
SNACK / TIME:								
LUNCH / TIME: **INSULIN:** **PRE SUGAR LEVEL:** **POST SUGAR LEVEL:**								
LUNCH TOTALS								
SNACK / TIME:								
DINNER / TIME: **INSULIN:** **PRE SUGAR LEVEL:** **POST SUGAR LEVEL:**								
DINNER TOTALS								
SNACK / TIME:								
DAILY TOTALS:								

VITAMINS / SUPPLEMENTS: _____

EXERCISE: _____

NOTES: _____

DAILY BLOOD SUGAR LOG

DAY/DATE: _____

WEIGHT: _____

MOOD/ENERGY: _____

	Glycemic index	Glycemic load	Calories (kcal)	Carbs (g)	Fiber (g)	Total sugar (g)	Added sugar (g)	Protein (g)
BREAKFAST / TIME: ___ **INSULIN:** ___ **PRE SUGAR LEVEL:** ___ **POST SUGAR LEVEL:** ___								
BREAKFAST TOTALS								
SNACK / TIME: ___								
LUNCH / TIME: ___ **INSULIN:** ___ **PRE SUGAR LEVEL:** ___ **POST SUGAR LEVEL:** ___								
LUNCH TOTALS								
SNACK / TIME: ___								
DINNER / TIME: ___ **INSULIN:** ___ **PRE SUGAR LEVEL:** ___ **POST SUGAR LEVEL:** ___								
DINNER TOTALS								
SNACK / TIME: ___								
DAILY TOTALS:								

VITAMINS / SUPPLEMENTS: _____

EXERCISE: _____

NOTES: _____

DAILY BLOOD SUGAR LOG

DAY/DATE: _____

WEIGHT: _____

MOOD/ENERGY: _____

	Glycemic index	Glycemic load	Calories (kcal)	Carbs (g)	Fiber (g)	Total sugar (g)	Added sugar (g)	Protein (g)
BREAKFAST / TIME: **INSULIN:** **PRE SUGAR LEVEL:** **POST SUGAR LEVEL:**								
BREAKFAST TOTALS								
SNACK / TIME:								
LUNCH / TIME: **INSULIN:** **PRE SUGAR LEVEL:** **POST SUGAR LEVEL:**								
LUNCH TOTALS								
SNACK / TIME:								
DINNER / TIME: **INSULIN:** **PRE SUGAR LEVEL:** **POST SUGAR LEVEL:**								
DINNER TOTALS								
SNACK / TIME:								
DAILY TOTALS:								

VITAMINS / SUPPLEMENTS:

EXERCISE:

NOTES:

DAILY BLOOD SUGAR LOG

DAY/DATE: _____

WEIGHT: _____

MOOD/ENERGY: _____

	Glycemic index	Glycemic load	Calories (kcal)	Carbs (g)	Fiber (g)	Total sugar (g)	Added sugar (g)	Protein (g)
BREAKFAST / TIME: INSULIN: PRE SUGAR LEVEL: POST SUGAR LEVEL:								
BREAKFAST TOTALS								
SNACK / TIME:								
LUNCH / TIME: INSULIN: PRE SUGAR LEVEL: POST SUGAR LEVEL:								
LUNCH TOTALS								
SNACK / TIME:								
DINNER / TIME: INSULIN: PRE SUGAR LEVEL: POST SUGAR LEVEL:								
DINNER TOTALS								
SNACK / TIME:								
DAILY TOTALS:								

VITAMINS / SUPPLEMENTS:

EXERCISE:

NOTES:

DAILY BLOOD SUGAR LOG

DAY / DATE: _____

WEIGHT: _____

MOOD / ENERGY: _____

	Glycemic index	Glycemic load	Calories (kcal)	Carbs (g)	Fiber (g)	Total sugar (g)	Added sugar (g)	Protein (g)
BREAKFAST / TIME: **INSULIN:** **PRE SUGAR LEVEL:** **POST SUGAR LEVEL:**								
BREAKFAST TOTALS								
SNACK / TIME:								
LUNCH / TIME: **INSULIN:** **PRE SUGAR LEVEL:** **POST SUGAR LEVEL:**								
LUNCH TOTALS								
SNACK / TIME:								
DINNER / TIME: **INSULIN:** **PRE SUGAR LEVEL:** **POST SUGAR LEVEL:**								
DINNER TOTALS								
SNACK / TIME:								
DAILY TOTALS:								

VITAMINS / SUPPLEMENTS:
_____

EXERCISE:
_____

NOTES:
_____

DAILY BLOOD SUGAR LOG

DAY/DATE: _____

WEIGHT: _____

MOOD/ENERGY: _____

	Glycemic index	Glycemic load	Calories (kcal)	Carbs (g)	Fiber (g)	Total sugar (g)	Added sugar (g)	Protein (g)
BREAKFAST / TIME: _____ **INSULIN:** _____ **PRE SUGAR LEVEL:** _____ **POST SUGAR LEVEL:** _____								
BREAKFAST TOTALS								
SNACK / TIME: _____								
LUNCH / TIME: _____ **INSULIN:** _____ **PRE SUGAR LEVEL:** _____ **POST SUGAR LEVEL:** _____								
LUNCH TOTALS								
SNACK / TIME: _____								
DINNER / TIME: _____ **INSULIN:** _____ **PRE SUGAR LEVEL:** _____ **POST SUGAR LEVEL:** _____								
DINNER TOTALS								
SNACK / TIME: _____								
DAILY TOTALS:								

VITAMINS / SUPPLEMENTS:

_____

EXERCISE:

_____

NOTES:

_____

DAILY BLOOD SUGAR LOG

DAY/DATE: _____

WEIGHT: _____

MOOD/ENERGY: _____

	Glycemic index	Glycemic load	Calories (kcal)	Carbs (g)	Fiber (g)	Total sugar (g)	Added sugar (g)	Protein (g)
BREAKFAST / TIME: INSULIN: PRE SUGAR LEVEL: POST SUGAR LEVEL:								
BREAKFAST TOTALS								
SNACK / TIME:								
LUNCH / TIME: INSULIN: PRE SUGAR LEVEL: POST SUGAR LEVEL:								
LUNCH TOTALS								
SNACK / TIME:								
DINNER / TIME: INSULIN: PRE SUGAR LEVEL: POST SUGAR LEVEL:								
DINNER TOTALS								
SNACK / TIME:								
DAILY TOTALS:								

VITAMINS / SUPPLEMENTS:

EXERCISE:

NOTES:

DAILY BLOOD SUGAR LOG

DAY/DATE: _____

WEIGHT: _____

MOOD/ENERGY: _____

	Glycemic index	Glycemic load	Calories (Kcal)	Carbs (g)	Fiber (g)	Total sugar (g)	Added sugar (g)	Protein (g)
BREAKFAST / TIME: INSULIN: PRE SUGAR LEVEL: POST SUGAR LEVEL:								
BREAKFAST TOTALS								
SNACK / TIME:								
LUNCH / TIME: INSULIN: PRE SUGAR LEVEL: POST SUGAR LEVEL:								
LUNCH TOTALS								
SNACK / TIME:								
DINNER / TIME: INSULIN: PRE SUGAR LEVEL: POST SUGAR LEVEL:								
DINNER TOTALS								
SNACK / TIME:								
DAILY TOTALS:								

VITAMINS / SUPPLEMENTS:
_____

EXERCISE:
_____

NOTES:
_____

DAILY BLOOD SUGAR LOG

DAY/DATE: _____

WEIGHT: _____

MOOD/ENERGY: _____

	Glycemic index	Glycemic load	Calories (kcal)	Carbs (g)	Fiber (g)	Total sugar (g)	Added sugar (g)	Protein (g)
BREAKFAST / TIME: _____ **INSULIN:** _____ **PRE SUGAR LEVEL:** _____ **POST SUGAR LEVEL:** _____								
BREAKFAST TOTALS								
SNACK / TIME: _____								
LUNCH / TIME: _____ **INSULIN:** _____ **PRE SUGAR LEVEL:** _____ **POST SUGAR LEVEL:** _____								
LUNCH TOTALS								
SNACK / TIME: _____								
DINNER / TIME: _____ **INSULIN:** _____ **PRE SUGAR LEVEL:** _____ **POST SUGAR LEVEL:** _____								
DINNER TOTALS								
SNACK / TIME: _____								
DAILY TOTALS:								

VITAMINS / SUPPLEMENTS:

EXERCISE:

NOTES:

DAILY BLOOD SUGAR LOG

DAY/DATE: _____

WEIGHT: _____

MOOD/ENERGY: _____

	Glycemic index	Glycemic load	Calories (kcal)	Carbs (g)	Fiber (g)	Total sugar (g)	Added sugar (g)	Protein (g)
BREAKFAST / TIME: **INSULIN:** **PRE SUGAR LEVEL:** **POST SUGAR LEVEL:**								
BREAKFAST TOTALS								
SNACK / TIME:								
LUNCH / TIME: **INSULIN:** **PRE SUGAR LEVEL:** **POST SUGAR LEVEL:**								
LUNCH TOTALS								
SNACK / TIME:								
DINNER / TIME: **INSULIN:** **PRE SUGAR LEVEL:** **POST SUGAR LEVEL:**								
DINNER TOTALS								
SNACK / TIME:								
DAILY TOTALS:								

VITAMINS / SUPPLEMENTS:
_____

EXERCISE:
_____

NOTES:
_____

DAILY BLOOD SUGAR LOG

DAY/DATE: _____

WEIGHT: _____

MOOD/ENERGY: _____

	Glycemic index	Glycemic load	Calories (kcal)	Carbs (g)	Fiber (g)	Total sugar (g)	Added sugar (g)	Protein (g)
BREAKFAST / TIME: __ **INSULIN:** __ **PRE SUGAR LEVEL:** __ **POST SUGAR LEVEL:** __								
BREAKFAST TOTALS								
SNACK / TIME:								
LUNCH / TIME: __ **INSULIN:** __ **PRE SUGAR LEVEL:** __ **POST SUGAR LEVEL:** __								
LUNCH TOTALS								
SNACK / TIME:								
DINNER / TIME: __ **INSULIN:** __ **PRE SUGAR LEVEL:** __ **POST SUGAR LEVEL:** __								
DINNER TOTALS								
SNACK / TIME:								
DAILY TOTALS:								

VITAMINS / SUPPLEMENTS:

_____

EXERCISE:

_____

NOTES:

_____

DAILY BLOOD SUGAR LOG

DAY/DATE: _____

WEIGHT: _____

MOOD/ENERGY: _____

	Glycemic index	Glycemic load	Calories (kcal)	Carbs (g)	Fiber (g)	Total sugar (g)	Added sugar (g)	Protein (g)
BREAKFAST / TIME: **INSULIN:** **PRE SUGAR LEVEL:** **POST SUGAR LEVEL:**								
BREAKFAST TOTALS								
SNACK / TIME:								
LUNCH / TIME: **INSULIN:** **PRE SUGAR LEVEL:** **POST SUGAR LEVEL:**								
LUNCH TOTALS								
SNACK / TIME:								
DINNER / TIME: **INSULIN:** **PRE SUGAR LEVEL:** **POST SUGAR LEVEL:**								
DINNER TOTALS								
SNACK / TIME:								
DAILY TOTALS:								

VITAMINS / SUPPLEMENTS:

EXERCISE:

NOTES:

DAILY BLOOD SUGAR LOG

DAY/DATE: _____

WEIGHT: _____

MOOD/ENERGY: _____

	Glycemic index	Glycemic load	Calories (kcal)	Carbs (g)	Fiber (g)	Total sugar (g)	Added sugar (g)	Protein (g)
BREAKFAST / TIME: **INSULIN:** **PRE SUGAR LEVEL:** **POST SUGAR LEVEL:**								
BREAKFAST TOTALS								
SNACK / TIME:								
LUNCH / TIME: **INSULIN:** **PRE SUGAR LEVEL:** **POST SUGAR LEVEL:**								
LUNCH TOTALS								
SNACK / TIME:								
DINNER / TIME: **INSULIN:** **PRE SUGAR LEVEL:** **POST SUGAR LEVEL:**								
DINNER TOTALS								
SNACK / TIME:								
DAILY TOTALS:								

VITAMINS / SUPPLEMENTS: _____

EXERCISE: _____

NOTES: _____

DAILY BLOOD SUGAR LOG

DAY/DATE: _____

WEIGHT: _____

MOOD/ENERGY: _____

	Glycemic index	Glycemic load	Calories (kcal)	Carbs (g)	Fiber (g)	Total sugar (g)	Added sugar (g)	Protein (g)
BREAKFAST / TIME: **INSULIN:** **PRE SUGAR LEVEL:** **POST SUGAR LEVEL:**								
BREAKFAST TOTALS								
SNACK / TIME:								
LUNCH / TIME: **INSULIN:** **PRE SUGAR LEVEL:** **POST SUGAR LEVEL:**								
LUNCH TOTALS								
SNACK / TIME:								
DINNER / TIME: **INSULIN:** **PRE SUGAR LEVEL:** **POST SUGAR LEVEL:**								
DINNER TOTALS								
SNACK / TIME:								
DAILY TOTALS:								

VITAMINS / SUPPLEMENTS:

EXERCISE:

NOTES:

DAILY BLOOD SUGAR LOG

DAY/DATE: _____

WEIGHT: _____

MOOD/ENERGY: _____

	Glycemic index	Glycemic load	Calories (kcal)	Carbs (g)	Fiber (g)	Total sugar (g)	Added sugar (g)	Protein (g)
BREAKFAST / TIME: INSULIN: PRE SUGAR LEVEL: POST SUGAR LEVEL:								
BREAKFAST TOTALS								
SNACK / TIME:								
LUNCH / TIME: INSULIN: PRE SUGAR LEVEL: POST SUGAR LEVEL:								
LUNCH TOTALS								
SNACK / TIME:								
DINNER / TIME: INSULIN: PRE SUGAR LEVEL: POST SUGAR LEVEL:								
DINNER TOTALS								
SNACK / TIME:								
DAILY TOTALS:								

VITAMINS / SUPPLEMENTS:

EXERCISE:

NOTES:

DAILY BLOOD SUGAR LOG

DAY/DATE: _____

WEIGHT: _____

MOOD/ENERGY: _____

	Glycemic index	Glycemic load	Calories (kcal)	Carbs (g)	Fiber (g)	Total sugar (g)	Added sugar (g)	Protein (g)
BREAKFAST / TIME: ____ **INSULIN:** ____ **PRE SUGAR LEVEL:** ____ **POST SUGAR LEVEL:** ____								
BREAKFAST TOTALS								
SNACK / TIME: ____								
LUNCH / TIME: ____ **INSULIN:** ____ **PRE SUGAR LEVEL:** ____ **POST SUGAR LEVEL:** ____								
LUNCH TOTALS								
SNACK / TIME: ____								
DINNER / TIME: ____ **INSULIN:** ____ **PRE SUGAR LEVEL:** ____ **POST SUGAR LEVEL:** ____								
DINNER TOTALS								
SNACK / TIME: ____								
DAILY TOTALS:								

VITAMINS / SUPPLEMENTS:

_____

EXERCISE:

_____

NOTES:

_____

DAILY BLOOD SUGAR LOG

DAY/DATE: _____

WEIGHT: _____

MOOD/ENERGY: _____

	Glycemic index	Glycemic load	Calories (kcal)	Carbs (g)	Fiber (g)	Total sugar (g)	Added sugar (g)	Protein (g)
BREAKFAST / TIME: ___ **INSULIN:** ___ **PRE SUGAR LEVEL:** ___ **POST SUGAR LEVEL:** ___								
BREAKFAST TOTALS								
SNACK / TIME:								
LUNCH / TIME: ___ **INSULIN:** ___ **PRE SUGAR LEVEL:** ___ **POST SUGAR LEVEL:** ___								
LUNCH TOTALS								
SNACK / TIME:								
DINNER / TIME: ___ **INSULIN:** ___ **PRE SUGAR LEVEL:** ___ **POST SUGAR LEVEL:** ___								
DINNER TOTALS								
SNACK / TIME:								
DAILY TOTALS:								

VITAMINS / SUPPLEMENTS: _____

EXERCISE: _____

NOTES: _____

DAILY BLOOD SUGAR LOG

DAY/DATE: _____

WEIGHT: _____

MOOD/ENERGY: _____

	Glycemic index	Glycemic load	Calories (kcal)	Carbs (g)	Fiber (g)	Total sugar (g)	Added sugar (g)	Protein (g)
BREAKFAST / TIME: ___ **INSULIN:** ___ **PRE SUGAR LEVEL:** ___ **POST SUGAR LEVEL:** ___								
BREAKFAST TOTALS								
SNACK / TIME: ___								
LUNCH / TIME: ___ **INSULIN:** ___ **PRE SUGAR LEVEL:** ___ **POST SUGAR LEVEL:** ___								
LUNCH TOTALS								
SNACK / TIME: ___								
DINNER / TIME: ___ **INSULIN:** ___ **PRE SUGAR LEVEL:** ___ **POST SUGAR LEVEL:** ___								
DINNER TOTALS								
SNACK / TIME: ___								
DAILY TOTALS:								

VITAMINS / SUPPLEMENTS:

EXERCISE:

NOTES:

DAILY BLOOD SUGAR LOG

DAY/DATE: _____

WEIGHT: _____

MOOD/ENERGY: _____

	Glycemic index	Glycemic load	Calories (kcal)	Carbs (g)	Fiber (g)	Total sugar (g)	Added sugar (g)	Protein (g)
BREAKFAST / TIME:	INSULIN:		PRE SUGAR LEVEL:			POST SUGAR LEVEL:		
BREAKFAST TOTALS								
SNACK / TIME:								
LUNCH / TIME:	INSULIN:		PRE SUGAR LEVEL:			POST SUGAR LEVEL:		
LUNCH TOTALS								
SNACK / TIME:								
DINNER / TIME:	INSULIN:		PRE SUGAR LEVEL:			POST SUGAR LEVEL:		
DINNER TOTALS								
SNACK / TIME:								
DAILY TOTALS:								

VITAMINS / SUPPLEMENTS:

EXERCISE:

NOTES:

DAILY BLOOD SUGAR LOG

DAY/DATE: _____

WEIGHT: _____

MOOD/ENERGY: _____

	Glycemic index	Glycemic load	Calories (kcal)	Carbs (g)	Fiber (g)	Total sugar (g)	Added sugar (g)	Protein (g)
BREAKFAST / TIME: ___ **INSULIN:** ___ **PRE SUGAR LEVEL:** ___ **POST SUGAR LEVEL:** ___								
BREAKFAST TOTALS								
SNACK / TIME: ___								
LUNCH / TIME: ___ **INSULIN:** ___ **PRE SUGAR LEVEL:** ___ **POST SUGAR LEVEL:** ___								
LUNCH TOTALS								
SNACK / TIME: ___								
DINNER / TIME: ___ **INSULIN:** ___ **PRE SUGAR LEVEL:** ___ **POST SUGAR LEVEL:** ___								
DINNER TOTALS								
SNACK / TIME: ___								
DAILY TOTALS:								

VITAMINS / SUPPLEMENTS:

EXERCISE:

NOTES:

DAILY BLOOD SUGAR LOG

DAY/DATE: _____

WEIGHT: _____

MOOD/ENERGY: _____

	Glycemic index	Glycemic load	Calories (kcal)	Carbs (g)	Fiber (g)	Total sugar (g)	Added sugar (g)	Protein (g)
BREAKFAST / TIME: INSULIN: PRE SUGAR LEVEL: POST SUGAR LEVEL:								
BREAKFAST TOTALS								
SNACK / TIME:								
LUNCH / TIME: INSULIN: PRE SUGAR LEVEL: POST SUGAR LEVEL:								
LUNCH TOTALS								
SNACK / TIME:								
DINNER / TIME: INSULIN: PRE SUGAR LEVEL: POST SUGAR LEVEL:								
DINNER TOTALS								
SNACK / TIME:								
DAILY TOTALS:								

VITAMINS / SUPPLEMENTS:

_____

EXERCISE:

_____

NOTES:

_____

DAILY BLOOD SUGAR LOG

DAY/DATE: _____

WEIGHT: _____

MOOD/ENERGY: _____

	Glycemic index	Glycemic load	Calories (kcal)	Carbs (g)	Fiber (g)	Total sugar (g)	Added sugar (g)	Protein (g)
BREAKFAST / TIME: INSULIN: PRE SUGAR LEVEL: POST SUGAR LEVEL:								
BREAKFAST TOTALS								
SNACK / TIME:								
LUNCH / TIME: INSULIN: PRE SUGAR LEVEL: POST SUGAR LEVEL:								
LUNCH TOTALS								
SNACK / TIME:								
DINNER / TIME: INSULIN: PRE SUGAR LEVEL: POST SUGAR LEVEL:								
DINNER TOTALS								
SNACK / TIME:								
DAILY TOTALS:								

VITAMINS / SUPPLEMENTS:

EXERCISE:

NOTES:

DAILY BLOOD SUGAR LOG

DAY/DATE: _____

WEIGHT: _____

MOOD/ENERGY: _____

	Glycemic index	Glycemic load	Calories (kcal)	Carbs (g)	Fiber (g)	Total sugar (g)	Added sugar (g)	Protein (g)
BREAKFAST / TIME: **INSULIN:** **PRE SUGAR LEVEL:** **POST SUGAR LEVEL:**								
BREAKFAST TOTALS								
SNACK / TIME:								
LUNCH / TIME: **INSULIN:** **PRE SUGAR LEVEL:** **POST SUGAR LEVEL:**								
LUNCH TOTALS								
SNACK / TIME:								
DINNER / TIME: **INSULIN:** **PRE SUGAR LEVEL:** **POST SUGAR LEVEL:**								
DINNER TOTALS								
SNACK / TIME:								
DAILY TOTALS:								

VITAMINS / SUPPLEMENTS:
_____

EXERCISE:
_____

NOTES:
_____

DAILY BLOOD SUGAR LOG

DAY/DATE: _____

WEIGHT: _____

MOOD/ENERGY: _____

	Glycemic index	Glycemic load	Calories (kcal)	Carbs (g)	Fiber (g)	Total sugar (g)	Added sugar (g)	Protein (g)
BREAKFAST / TIME: **INSULIN:** **PRE SUGAR LEVEL:** **POST SUGAR LEVEL:**								
BREAKFAST TOTALS								
SNACK / TIME:								
LUNCH / TIME: **INSULIN:** **PRE SUGAR LEVEL:** **POST SUGAR LEVEL:**								
LUNCH TOTALS								
SNACK / TIME:								
DINNER / TIME: **INSULIN:** **PRE SUGAR LEVEL:** **POST SUGAR LEVEL:**								
DINNER TOTALS								
SNACK / TIME:								
DAILY TOTALS:								

VITAMINS / SUPPLEMENTS:

EXERCISE:

NOTES:

DAILY BLOOD SUGAR LOG

DAY/DATE: _____

WEIGHT: _____

MOOD/ENERGY: _____

	Glycemic index	Glycemic load	Calories (Kcal)	Carbs (g)	Fiber (g)	Total sugar (g)	Added sugar (g)	Protein (g)
BREAKFAST / TIME: **INSULIN:** **PRE SUGAR LEVEL:** **POST SUGAR LEVEL:**								
BREAKFAST TOTALS								
SNACK / TIME:								
LUNCH / TIME: **INSULIN:** **PRE SUGAR LEVEL:** **POST SUGAR LEVEL:**								
LUNCH TOTALS								
SNACK / TIME:								
DINNER / TIME: **INSULIN:** **PRE SUGAR LEVEL:** **POST SUGAR LEVEL:**								
DINNER TOTALS								
SNACK / TIME:								
DAILY TOTALS:								

VITAMINS / SUPPLEMENTS:

EXERCISE:

NOTES:

DAILY BLOOD SUGAR LOG

DAY / DATE: _____

WEIGHT: _____

MOOD / ENERGY: _____

	Glycemic index	Glycemic load	Calories (kcal)	Carbs (g)	Fiber (g)	Total sugar (g)	Added sugar (g)	Protein (g)
BREAKFAST / TIME: **INSULIN:** **PRE SUGAR LEVEL:** **POST SUGAR LEVEL:**								
BREAKFAST TOTALS								
SNACK / TIME:								
LUNCH / TIME: **INSULIN:** **PRE SUGAR LEVEL:** **POST SUGAR LEVEL:**								
LUNCH TOTALS								
SNACK / TIME:								
DINNER / TIME: **INSULIN:** **PRE SUGAR LEVEL:** **POST SUGAR LEVEL:**								
DINNER TOTALS								
SNACK / TIME:								
DAILY TOTALS:								

VITAMINS / SUPPLEMENTS:

EXERCISE:

NOTES:

DAILY BLOOD SUGAR LOG

DAY/DATE: _____

WEIGHT: _____

MOOD/ENERGY: _____

	Glycemic index	Glycemic load	Calories (kcal)	Carbs (g)	Fiber (g)	Total sugar (g)	Added sugar (g)	Protein (g)
BREAKFAST / TIME: **INSULIN:** **PRE SUGAR LEVEL:** **POST SUGAR LEVEL:**								
BREAKFAST TOTALS								
SNACK / TIME:								
LUNCH / TIME: **INSULIN:** **PRE SUGAR LEVEL:** **POST SUGAR LEVEL:**								
LUNCH TOTALS								
SNACK / TIME:								
DINNER / TIME: **INSULIN:** **PRE SUGAR LEVEL:** **POST SUGAR LEVEL:**								
DINNER TOTALS								
SNACK / TIME:								
DAILY TOTALS:								

VITAMINS / SUPPLEMENTS:

EXERCISE:

NOTES:

DAILY BLOOD SUGAR LOG

DAY/DATE: _____

WEIGHT: _____

MOOD/ENERGY: _____

	Glycemic index	Glycemic load	Calories (kcal)	Carbs (g)	Fiber (g)	Total sugar (g)	Added sugar (g)	Protein (g)
BREAKFAST / TIME: **INSULIN:** **PRE SUGAR LEVEL:** **POST SUGAR LEVEL:**								
BREAKFAST TOTALS								
SNACK / TIME:								
LUNCH / TIME: **INSULIN:** **PRE SUGAR LEVEL:** **POST SUGAR LEVEL:**								
LUNCH TOTALS								
SNACK / TIME:								
DINNER / TIME: **INSULIN:** **PRE SUGAR LEVEL:** **POST SUGAR LEVEL:**								
DINNER TOTALS								
SNACK / TIME:								
DAILY TOTALS:								

VITAMINS / SUPPLEMENTS:

EXERCISE:

NOTES:

DAILY BLOOD SUGAR LOG

DAY/DATE: _____

WEIGHT: _____

MOOD/ENERGY: _____

	Glycemic index	Glycemic load	Calories (kcal)	Carbs (g)	Fiber (g)	Total sugar (g)	Added sugar (g)	Protein (g)
BREAKFAST / TIME: INSULIN: PRE SUGAR LEVEL: POST SUGAR LEVEL:								
BREAKFAST TOTALS								
SNACK / TIME:								
LUNCH / TIME: INSULIN: PRE SUGAR LEVEL: POST SUGAR LEVEL:								
LUNCH TOTALS								
SNACK / TIME:								
DINNER / TIME: INSULIN: PRE SUGAR LEVEL: POST SUGAR LEVEL:								
DINNER TOTALS								
SNACK / TIME:								
DAILY TOTALS:								

VITAMINS / SUPPLEMENTS:
_____

EXERCISE:
_____
_____

NOTES:
_____
_____

DAILY BLOOD SUGAR LOG

DAY/DATE: _____

WEIGHT: _____

MOOD/ENERGY: _____

	Glycemic index	Glycemic load	Calories (kcal)	Carbs (g)	Fiber (g)	Total sugar (g)	Added sugar (g)	Protein (g)
BREAKFAST / TIME: INSULIN: PRE SUGAR LEVEL: POST SUGAR LEVEL:								
BREAKFAST TOTALS								
SNACK / TIME:								
LUNCH / TIME: INSULIN: PRE SUGAR LEVEL: POST SUGAR LEVEL:								
LUNCH TOTALS								
SNACK / TIME:								
DINNER / TIME: INSULIN: PRE SUGAR LEVEL: POST SUGAR LEVEL:								
DINNER TOTALS								
SNACK / TIME:								
DAILY TOTALS:								

VITAMINS / SUPPLEMENTS: _____
_____

EXERCISE: _____
_____

NOTES: _____

DAILY BLOOD SUGAR LOG

DAY/DATE: _____

WEIGHT: _____

MOOD/ENERGY: _____

	Glycemic index	Glycemic load	Calories (kcal)	Carbs (g)	Fiber (g)	Total sugar (g)	Added sugar (g)	Protein (g)
BREAKFAST / TIME: INSULIN: PRE SUGAR LEVEL: POST SUGAR LEVEL:								
BREAKFAST TOTALS								
SNACK / TIME:								
LUNCH / TIME: INSULIN: PRE SUGAR LEVEL: POST SUGAR LEVEL:								
LUNCH TOTALS								
SNACK / TIME:								
DINNER / TIME: INSULIN: PRE SUGAR LEVEL: POST SUGAR LEVEL:								
DINNER TOTALS								
SNACK / TIME:								
DAILY TOTALS:								

VITAMINS / SUPPLEMENTS: _____

EXERCISE: _____

NOTES: _____

DAILY BLOOD SUGAR LOG

DAY/DATE: _____

WEIGHT: _____

MOOD/ENERGY: _____

	Glycemic index	Glycemic load	Calories (kcal)	Carbs (g)	Fiber (g)	Total sugar (g)	Added sugar (g)	Protein (g)
BREAKFAST / TIME: ___ **INSULIN:** ___ **PRE SUGAR LEVEL:** ___ **POST SUGAR LEVEL:** ___								
BREAKFAST TOTALS								
SNACK / TIME: ___								
LUNCH / TIME: ___ **INSULIN:** ___ **PRE SUGAR LEVEL:** ___ **POST SUGAR LEVEL:** ___								
LUNCH TOTALS								
SNACK / TIME: ___								
DINNER / TIME: ___ **INSULIN:** ___ **PRE SUGAR LEVEL:** ___ **POST SUGAR LEVEL:** ___								
DINNER TOTALS								
SNACK / TIME: ___								
DAILY TOTALS:								

VITAMINS / SUPPLEMENTS:

_____

EXERCISE:

_____

NOTES:

_____

DAILY BLOOD SUGAR LOG

DAY/DATE: _____

WEIGHT: _____

MOOD/ENERGY: _____

	Glycemic index	Glycemic load	Calories (kcal)	Carbs (g)	Fiber (g)	Total sugar (g)	Added sugar (g)	Protein (g)
BREAKFAST / TIME: ___ **INSULIN:** ___ **PRE SUGAR LEVEL:** ___ **POST SUGAR LEVEL:** ___								
BREAKFAST TOTALS								
SNACK / TIME: ___								
LUNCH / TIME: ___ **INSULIN:** ___ **PRE SUGAR LEVEL:** ___ **POST SUGAR LEVEL:** ___								
LUNCH TOTALS								
SNACK / TIME: ___								
DINNER / TIME: ___ **INSULIN:** ___ **PRE SUGAR LEVEL:** ___ **POST SUGAR LEVEL:** ___								
DINNER TOTALS								
SNACK / TIME: ___								
DAILY TOTALS:								

VITAMINS / SUPPLEMENTS: _____

EXERCISE: _____

NOTES: _____

DAILY BLOOD SUGAR LOG

DAY/DATE: _____

WEIGHT: _____

MOOD/ENERGY: _____

	Glycemic index	Glycemic load	Calories (Kcal)	Carbs (g)	Fiber (g)	Total sugar (g)	Added sugar (g)	Protein (g)
BREAKFAST / TIME: INSULIN: PRE SUGAR LEVEL: POST SUGAR LEVEL:								
BREAKFAST TOTALS								
SNACK / TIME:								
LUNCH / TIME: INSULIN: PRE SUGAR LEVEL: POST SUGAR LEVEL:								
LUNCH TOTALS								
SNACK / TIME:								
DINNER / TIME: INSULIN: PRE SUGAR LEVEL: POST SUGAR LEVEL:								
DINNER TOTALS								
SNACK / TIME:								
DAILY TOTALS:								

VITAMINS / SUPPLEMENTS: _____

EXERCISE: _____

NOTES: _____

DAILY BLOOD SUGAR LOG

DAY/DATE: _____

WEIGHT: _____

MOOD/ENERGY: _____

	Glycemic index	Glycemic load	Calories (kcal)	Carbs (g)	Fiber (g)	Total sugar (g)	Added sugar (g)	Protein (g)
BREAKFAST / TIME: — INSULIN: — PRE SUGAR LEVEL: — POST SUGAR LEVEL:								
BREAKFAST TOTALS								
SNACK / TIME:								
LUNCH / TIME: — INSULIN: — PRE SUGAR LEVEL: — POST SUGAR LEVEL:								
LUNCH TOTALS								
SNACK / TIME:								
DINNER / TIME: — INSULIN: — PRE SUGAR LEVEL: — POST SUGAR LEVEL:								
DINNER TOTALS								
SNACK / TIME:								
DAILY TOTALS:								

VITAMINS / SUPPLEMENTS:
_____

EXERCISE:
_____

NOTES:
_____

DAILY BLOOD SUGAR LOG

DAY/DATE: _____

WEIGHT: _____

MOOD/ENERGY: _____

	Glycemic index	Glycemic load	Calories (kcal)	Carbs (g)	Fiber (g)	Total sugar (g)	Added sugar (g)	Protein (g)
BREAKFAST / TIME: INSULIN: PRE SUGAR LEVEL: POST SUGAR LEVEL:								
BREAKFAST TOTALS								
SNACK / TIME:								
LUNCH / TIME: INSULIN: PRE SUGAR LEVEL: POST SUGAR LEVEL:								
LUNCH TOTALS								
SNACK / TIME:								
DINNER / TIME: INSULIN: PRE SUGAR LEVEL: POST SUGAR LEVEL:								
DINNER TOTALS								
SNACK / TIME:								
DAILY TOTALS:								

VITAMINS / SUPPLEMENTS:

_____

EXERCISE:

_____

NOTES:

_____

DAILY BLOOD SUGAR LOG

DAY/DATE: _____

WEIGHT: _____

MOOD/ENERGY: _____

	Glycemic index	Glycemic load	Calories (kcal)	Carbs (g)	Fiber (g)	Total sugar (g)	Added sugar (g)	Protein (g)
BREAKFAST / TIME:　INSULIN:　PRE SUGAR LEVEL:　POST SUGAR LEVEL:								
BREAKFAST TOTALS								
SNACK / TIME:								
LUNCH / TIME:　INSULIN:　PRE SUGAR LEVEL:　POST SUGAR LEVEL:								
LUNCH TOTALS								
SNACK / TIME:								
DINNER / TIME:　INSULIN:　PRE SUGAR LEVEL:　POST SUGAR LEVEL:								
DINNER TOTALS								
SNACK / TIME:								
DAILY TOTALS:								

VITAMINS / SUPPLEMENTS:

EXERCISE:

NOTES:

DAILY BLOOD SUGAR LOG

DAY/DATE: _____

WEIGHT: _____

MOOD/ENERGY: _____

	Glycemic index	Glycemic load	Calories (Kcal)	Carbs (g)	Fiber (g)	Total sugar (g)	Added sugar (g)	Protein (g)
BREAKFAST / TIME: — INSULIN: — PRE SUGAR LEVEL: — POST SUGAR LEVEL:								
BREAKFAST TOTALS								
SNACK / TIME:								
LUNCH / TIME: — INSULIN: — PRE SUGAR LEVEL: — POST SUGAR LEVEL:								
LUNCH TOTALS								
SNACK / TIME:								
DINNER / TIME: — INSULIN: — PRE SUGAR LEVEL: — POST SUGAR LEVEL:								
DINNER TOTALS								
SNACK / TIME:								
DAILY TOTALS:								

VITAMINS / SUPPLEMENTS: _____

EXERCISE: _____

NOTES: _____

DAILY BLOOD SUGAR LOG

DAY/DATE: _____

WEIGHT: _____

MOOD/ENERGY: _____

	Glycemic index	Glycemic load	Calories (kcal)	Carbs (g)	Fiber (g)	Total sugar (g)	Added sugar (g)	Protein (g)
BREAKFAST / TIME: INSULIN: PRE SUGAR LEVEL: POST SUGAR LEVEL:								
BREAKFAST TOTALS								
SNACK / TIME:								
LUNCH / TIME: INSULIN: PRE SUGAR LEVEL: POST SUGAR LEVEL:								
LUNCH TOTALS								
SNACK / TIME:								
DINNER / TIME: INSULIN: PRE SUGAR LEVEL: POST SUGAR LEVEL:								
DINNER TOTALS								
SNACK / TIME:								
DAILY TOTALS:								

VITAMINS / SUPPLEMENTS:

EXERCISE:

NOTES:

DAILY BLOOD SUGAR LOG

DAY/DATE: _____

WEIGHT: _____

MOOD/ENERGY: _____

	Glycemic index	Glycemic load	Calories (kcal)	Carbs (g)	Fiber (g)	Total sugar (g)	Added sugar (g)	Protein (g)
BREAKFAST / TIME: ____ **INSULIN:** ____ **PRE SUGAR LEVEL:** ____ **POST SUGAR LEVEL:** ____								
BREAKFAST TOTALS								
SNACK / TIME: ____								
LUNCH / TIME: ____ **INSULIN:** ____ **PRE SUGAR LEVEL:** ____ **POST SUGAR LEVEL:** ____								
LUNCH TOTALS								
SNACK / TIME: ____								
DINNER / TIME: ____ **INSULIN:** ____ **PRE SUGAR LEVEL:** ____ **POST SUGAR LEVEL:** ____								
DINNER TOTALS								
SNACK / TIME: ____								
DAILY TOTALS:								

VITAMINS / SUPPLEMENTS:

_____

EXERCISE:

_____

NOTES:

_____

DAILY BLOOD SUGAR LOG

DAY/DATE: _____

WEIGHT: _____

MOOD/ENERGY: _____

	Glycemic index	Glycemic load	Calories (kcal)	Carbs (g)	Fiber (g)	Total sugar (g)	Added sugar (g)	Protein (g)
BREAKFAST / TIME: **INSULIN:** **PRE SUGAR LEVEL:** **POST SUGAR LEVEL:**								
BREAKFAST TOTALS								
SNACK / TIME:								
LUNCH / TIME: **INSULIN:** **PRE SUGAR LEVEL:** **POST SUGAR LEVEL:**								
LUNCH TOTALS								
SNACK / TIME:								
DINNER / TIME: **INSULIN:** **PRE SUGAR LEVEL:** **POST SUGAR LEVEL:**								
DINNER TOTALS								
SNACK / TIME:								
DAILY TOTALS:								

VITAMINS / SUPPLEMENTS: _____

EXERCISE: _____

NOTES: _____

DAILY BLOOD SUGAR LOG

DAY/DATE: _____

WEIGHT: _____

MOOD/ENERGY: _____

	Glycemic index	Glycemic load	Calories (kcal)	Carbs (g)	Fiber (g)	Total sugar (g)	Added sugar (g)	Protein (g)
BREAKFAST / TIME: INSULIN: PRE SUGAR LEVEL: POST SUGAR LEVEL:								
BREAKFAST TOTALS								
SNACK / TIME:								
LUNCH / TIME: INSULIN: PRE SUGAR LEVEL: POST SUGAR LEVEL:								
LUNCH TOTALS								
SNACK / TIME:								
DINNER / TIME: INSULIN: PRE SUGAR LEVEL: POST SUGAR LEVEL:								
DINNER TOTALS								
SNACK / TIME:								
DAILY TOTALS:								

VITAMINS / SUPPLEMENTS:

EXERCISE:

NOTES:

DAILY BLOOD SUGAR LOG

DAY/DATE: _____

WEIGHT: _____

MOOD/ENERGY: _____

	Glycemic index	Glycemic load	Calories (kcal)	Carbs (g)	Fiber (g)	Total sugar (g)	Added sugar (g)	Protein (g)
BREAKFAST / TIME: INSULIN: PRE SUGAR LEVEL: POST SUGAR LEVEL:								
BREAKFAST TOTALS								
SNACK / TIME:								
LUNCH / TIME: INSULIN: PRE SUGAR LEVEL: POST SUGAR LEVEL:								
LUNCH TOTALS								
SNACK / TIME:								
DINNER / TIME: INSULIN: PRE SUGAR LEVEL: POST SUGAR LEVEL:								
DINNER TOTALS								
SNACK / TIME:								
DAILY TOTALS:								

VITAMINS / SUPPLEMENTS:
_____

EXERCISE:
_____

NOTES:
_____

DAILY BLOOD SUGAR LOG

DAY/DATE: _____

WEIGHT: _____

MOOD/ENERGY: _____

	Glycemic index	Glycemic load	Calories (kcal)	Carbs (g)	Fiber (g)	Total sugar (g)	Added sugar (g)	Protein (g)
BREAKFAST / TIME: ___ **INSULIN:** ___ **PRE SUGAR LEVEL:** ___ **POST SUGAR LEVEL:** ___								
BREAKFAST TOTALS								
SNACK / TIME: ___								
LUNCH / TIME: ___ **INSULIN:** ___ **PRE SUGAR LEVEL:** ___ **POST SUGAR LEVEL:** ___								
LUNCH TOTALS								
SNACK / TIME: ___								
DINNER / TIME: ___ **INSULIN:** ___ **PRE SUGAR LEVEL:** ___ **POST SUGAR LEVEL:** ___								
DINNER TOTALS								
SNACK / TIME: ___								
DAILY TOTALS:								

VITAMINS / SUPPLEMENTS: _____

EXERCISE: _____

NOTES: _____

DAILY BLOOD SUGAR LOG

DAY/DATE: _____

WEIGHT: _____

MOOD/ENERGY: _____

	Glycemic index	Glycemic load	Calories (kcal)	Carbs (g)	Fiber (g)	Total sugar (g)	Added sugar (g)	Protein (g)
BREAKFAST / TIME: ___ **INSULIN:** ___ **PRE SUGAR LEVEL:** ___ **POST SUGAR LEVEL:** ___								
BREAKFAST TOTALS								
SNACK / TIME: ___								
LUNCH / TIME: ___ **INSULIN:** ___ **PRE SUGAR LEVEL:** ___ **POST SUGAR LEVEL:** ___								
LUNCH TOTALS								
SNACK / TIME: ___								
DINNER / TIME: ___ **INSULIN:** ___ **PRE SUGAR LEVEL:** ___ **POST SUGAR LEVEL:** ___								
DINNER TOTALS								
SNACK / TIME: ___								
DAILY TOTALS:								

VITAMINS / SUPPLEMENTS:

EXERCISE:

NOTES:

DAILY BLOOD SUGAR LOG

DAY/DATE: _____

WEIGHT: _____

MOOD/ENERGY: _____

	Glycemic index	Glycemic load	Calories (kcal)	Carbs (g)	Fiber (g)	Total sugar (g)	Added sugar (g)	Protein (g)
BREAKFAST / TIME: _____ **INSULIN:** _____ **PRE SUGAR LEVEL:** _____ **POST SUGAR LEVEL:** _____								
BREAKFAST TOTALS								
SNACK / TIME: _____								
LUNCH / TIME: _____ **INSULIN:** _____ **PRE SUGAR LEVEL:** _____ **POST SUGAR LEVEL:** _____								
LUNCH TOTALS								
SNACK / TIME: _____								
DINNER / TIME: _____ **INSULIN:** _____ **PRE SUGAR LEVEL:** _____ **POST SUGAR LEVEL:** _____								
DINNER TOTALS								
SNACK / TIME: _____								
DAILY TOTALS:								

VITAMINS / SUPPLEMENTS:
_____

EXERCISE:
_____

NOTES:
_____

DAILY BLOOD SUGAR LOG

DAY/DATE: _____

WEIGHT: _____

MOOD/ENERGY: _____

	Glycemic index	Glycemic load	Calories (kcal)	Carbs (g)	Fiber (g)	Total sugar (g)	Added sugar (g)	Protein (g)
BREAKFAST / TIME: ___ **INSULIN:** ___ **PRE SUGAR LEVEL:** ___ **POST SUGAR LEVEL:** ___								
BREAKFAST TOTALS								
SNACK / TIME: ___								
LUNCH / TIME: ___ **INSULIN:** ___ **PRE SUGAR LEVEL:** ___ **POST SUGAR LEVEL:** ___								
LUNCH TOTALS								
SNACK / TIME: ___								
DINNER / TIME: ___ **INSULIN:** ___ **PRE SUGAR LEVEL:** ___ **POST SUGAR LEVEL:** ___								
DINNER TOTALS								
SNACK / TIME: ___								
DAILY TOTALS:								

VITAMINS / SUPPLEMENTS:
_____

EXERCISE:
_____

NOTES:
_____

DAILY BLOOD SUGAR LOG

DAY / DATE: _____

WEIGHT: _____

MOOD / ENERGY: _____

	Glycemic index	Glycemic load	Calories (kcal)	Carbs (g)	Fiber (g)	Total sugar (g)	Added sugar (g)	Protein (g)
BREAKFAST / TIME: INSULIN: PRE SUGAR LEVEL: POST SUGAR LEVEL:								
BREAKFAST TOTALS								
SNACK / TIME:								
LUNCH / TIME: INSULIN: PRE SUGAR LEVEL: POST SUGAR LEVEL:								
LUNCH TOTALS								
SNACK / TIME:								
DINNER / TIME: INSULIN: PRE SUGAR LEVEL: POST SUGAR LEVEL:								
DINNER TOTALS								
SNACK / TIME:								
DAILY TOTALS:								

VITAMINS / SUPPLEMENTS: _____

EXERCISE: _____

NOTES: _____

DAILY BLOOD SUGAR LOG

DAY/DATE: _____

WEIGHT: _____

MOOD/ENERGY: _____

	Glycemic index	Glycemic load	Calories (kcal)	Carbs (g)	Fiber (g)	Total sugar (g)	Added sugar (g)	Protein (g)
BREAKFAST / TIME: — **INSULIN:** — **PRE SUGAR LEVEL:** — **POST SUGAR LEVEL:**								
BREAKFAST TOTALS								
SNACK / TIME:								
LUNCH / TIME: — **INSULIN:** — **PRE SUGAR LEVEL:** — **POST SUGAR LEVEL:**								
LUNCH TOTALS								
SNACK / TIME:								
DINNER / TIME: — **INSULIN:** — **PRE SUGAR LEVEL:** — **POST SUGAR LEVEL:**								
DINNER TOTALS								
SNACK / TIME:								
DAILY TOTALS:								

VITAMINS / SUPPLEMENTS:

EXERCISE:

NOTES:

DAILY BLOOD SUGAR LOG

DAY/DATE: _____

WEIGHT: _____

MOOD/ENERGY: _____

	Glycemic index	Glycemic load	Calories (kcal)	Carbs (g)	Fiber (g)	Total sugar (g)	Added sugar (g)	Protein (g)
BREAKFAST / TIME: **INSULIN:** **PRE SUGAR LEVEL:** **POST SUGAR LEVEL:**								
BREAKFAST TOTALS								
SNACK / TIME:								
LUNCH / TIME: **INSULIN:** **PRE SUGAR LEVEL:** **POST SUGAR LEVEL:**								
LUNCH TOTALS								
SNACK / TIME:								
DINNER / TIME: **INSULIN:** **PRE SUGAR LEVEL:** **POST SUGAR LEVEL:**								
DINNER TOTALS								
SNACK / TIME:								
DAILY TOTALS:								

VITAMINS / SUPPLEMENTS:
_____

EXERCISE:
_____

NOTES:
_____

DAILY BLOOD SUGAR LOG

DAY/DATE: _____

WEIGHT: _____

MOOD/ENERGY: _____

	Glycemic index	Glycemic load	Calories (kcal)	Carbs (g)	Fiber (g)	Total sugar (g)	Added sugar (g)	Protein (g)
BREAKFAST / TIME: ___ **INSULIN:** ___ **PRE SUGAR LEVEL:** ___ **POST SUGAR LEVEL:** ___								
BREAKFAST TOTALS								
SNACK / TIME: ___								
LUNCH / TIME: ___ **INSULIN:** ___ **PRE SUGAR LEVEL:** ___ **POST SUGAR LEVEL:** ___								
LUNCH TOTALS								
SNACK / TIME: ___								
DINNER / TIME: ___ **INSULIN:** ___ **PRE SUGAR LEVEL:** ___ **POST SUGAR LEVEL:** ___								
DINNER TOTALS								
SNACK / TIME: ___								
DAILY TOTALS:								

VITAMINS / SUPPLEMENTS:

_____

EXERCISE:

_____

_____

NOTES:

_____

_____

87

DAILY BLOOD SUGAR LOG

DAY/DATE: _____

WEIGHT: _____

MOOD/ENERGY: _____

	Glycemic index	Glycemic load	Calories (kcal)	Carbs (g)	Fiber (g)	Total sugar (g)	Added sugar (g)	Protein (g)
BREAKFAST / TIME: ___ **INSULIN:** ___ **PRE SUGAR LEVEL:** ___ **POST SUGAR LEVEL:** ___								
BREAKFAST TOTALS								
SNACK / TIME: ___								
LUNCH / TIME: ___ **INSULIN:** ___ **PRE SUGAR LEVEL:** ___ **POST SUGAR LEVEL:** ___								
LUNCH TOTALS								
SNACK / TIME: ___								
DINNER / TIME: ___ **INSULIN:** ___ **PRE SUGAR LEVEL:** ___ **POST SUGAR LEVEL:** ___								
DINNER TOTALS								
SNACK / TIME: ___								
DAILY TOTALS:								

VITAMINS / SUPPLEMENTS:

EXERCISE:

NOTES:

DAILY BLOOD SUGAR LOG

DAY/DATE: _____

WEIGHT: _____

MOOD/ENERGY: _____

	Glycemic index	Glycemic load	Calories (Kcal)	Carbs (g)	Fiber (g)	Total sugar (g)	Added sugar (g)	Protein (g)
BREAKFAST / TIME: **INSULIN:** **PRE SUGAR LEVEL:** **POST SUGAR LEVEL:**								
BREAKFAST TOTALS								
SNACK / TIME:								
LUNCH / TIME: **INSULIN:** **PRE SUGAR LEVEL:** **POST SUGAR LEVEL:**								
LUNCH TOTALS								
SNACK / TIME:								
DINNER / TIME: **INSULIN:** **PRE SUGAR LEVEL:** **POST SUGAR LEVEL:**								
DINNER TOTALS								
SNACK / TIME:								
DAILY TOTALS:								

VITAMINS / SUPPLEMENTS:

EXERCISE:

NOTES:

DAILY BLOOD SUGAR LOG

DAY/DATE: _____

WEIGHT: _____

MOOD/ENERGY: _____

	Glycemic index	Glycemic load	Calories (kcal)	Carbs (g)	Fiber (g)	Total sugar (g)	Added sugar (g)	Protein (g)
BREAKFAST / TIME: **INSULIN:** **PRE SUGAR LEVEL:** **POST SUGAR LEVEL:**								
BREAKFAST TOTALS								
SNACK / TIME:								
LUNCH / TIME: **INSULIN:** **PRE SUGAR LEVEL:** **POST SUGAR LEVEL:**								
LUNCH TOTALS								
SNACK / TIME:								
DINNER / TIME: **INSULIN:** **PRE SUGAR LEVEL:** **POST SUGAR LEVEL:**								
DINNER TOTALS								
SNACK / TIME:								
DAILY TOTALS:								

VITAMINS / SUPPLEMENTS:

EXERCISE:

NOTES:

DAILY BLOOD SUGAR LOG

DAY/DATE: _____

WEIGHT: _____

MOOD/ENERGY: _____

	Glycemic index	Glycemic load	Calories (kcal)	Carbs (g)	Fiber (g)	Total sugar (g)	Added sugar (g)	Protein (g)
BREAKFAST / TIME: INSULIN: PRE SUGAR LEVEL: POST SUGAR LEVEL:								
BREAKFAST TOTALS								
SNACK / TIME:								
LUNCH / TIME: INSULIN: PRE SUGAR LEVEL: POST SUGAR LEVEL:								
LUNCH TOTALS								
SNACK / TIME:								
DINNER / TIME: INSULIN: PRE SUGAR LEVEL: POST SUGAR LEVEL:								
DINNER TOTALS								
SNACK / TIME:								
DAILY TOTALS:								

VITAMINS / SUPPLEMENTS:

_____

EXERCISE:

_____

NOTES:

_____

DAILY BLOOD SUGAR LOG

DAY/DATE: _____

WEIGHT: _____

MOOD/ENERGY: _____

	Glycemic index	Glycemic load	Calories (kcal)	Carbs (g)	Fiber (g)	Total sugar (g)	Added sugar (g)	Protein (g)
BREAKFAST / TIME: _____ **INSULIN:** _____ **PRE SUGAR LEVEL:** _____ **POST SUGAR LEVEL:** _____								
BREAKFAST TOTALS								
SNACK / TIME: _____								
LUNCH / TIME: _____ **INSULIN:** _____ **PRE SUGAR LEVEL:** _____ **POST SUGAR LEVEL:** _____								
LUNCH TOTALS								
SNACK / TIME: _____								
DINNER / TIME: _____ **INSULIN:** _____ **PRE SUGAR LEVEL:** _____ **POST SUGAR LEVEL:** _____								
DINNER TOTALS								
SNACK / TIME: _____								
DAILY TOTALS:								

VITAMINS / SUPPLEMENTS:

EXERCISE:

NOTES:

DAILY BLOOD SUGAR LOG

DAY/DATE: _____

WEIGHT: _____

MOOD/ENERGY: _____

	Glycemic index	Glycemic load	Calories (kcal)	Carbs (g)	Fiber (g)	Total sugar (g)	Added sugar (g)	Protein (g)
BREAKFAST / TIME: ___ **INSULIN:** ___ **PRE SUGAR LEVEL:** ___ **POST SUGAR LEVEL:** ___								
BREAKFAST TOTALS								
SNACK / TIME: ___								
LUNCH / TIME: ___ **INSULIN:** ___ **PRE SUGAR LEVEL:** ___ **POST SUGAR LEVEL:** ___								
LUNCH TOTALS								
SNACK / TIME: ___								
DINNER / TIME: ___ **INSULIN:** ___ **PRE SUGAR LEVEL:** ___ **POST SUGAR LEVEL:** ___								
DINNER TOTALS								
SNACK / TIME: ___								
DAILY TOTALS:								

VITAMINS / SUPPLEMENTS:
_____

EXERCISE:
_____

NOTES:
_____

DAILY BLOOD SUGAR LOG

DAY/DATE: _____

WEIGHT: _____

MOOD/ENERGY: _____

	Glycemic index	Glycemic load	Calories (kcal)	Carbs (g)	Fiber (g)	Total sugar (g)	Added sugar (g)	Protein (g)
BREAKFAST / TIME: ___ **INSULIN:** ___ **PRE SUGAR LEVEL:** ___ **POST SUGAR LEVEL:** ___								
BREAKFAST TOTALS								
SNACK / TIME: ___								
LUNCH / TIME: ___ **INSULIN:** ___ **PRE SUGAR LEVEL:** ___ **POST SUGAR LEVEL:** ___								
LUNCH TOTALS								
SNACK / TIME: ___								
DINNER / TIME: ___ **INSULIN:** ___ **PRE SUGAR LEVEL:** ___ **POST SUGAR LEVEL:** ___								
DINNER TOTALS								
SNACK / TIME: ___								
DAILY TOTALS:								

VITAMINS / SUPPLEMENTS:

EXERCISE:

NOTES:

DAILY BLOOD SUGAR LOG

DAY/DATE: _____

WEIGHT: _____

MOOD/ENERGY: _____

	Glycemic index	Glycemic load	Calories (kcal)	Carbs (g)	Fiber (g)	Total sugar (g)	Added sugar (g)	Protein (g)
BREAKFAST / TIME: __ **INSULIN:** __ **PRE SUGAR LEVEL:** __ **POST SUGAR LEVEL:** __								
BREAKFAST TOTALS								
SNACK / TIME: __								
LUNCH / TIME: __ **INSULIN:** __ **PRE SUGAR LEVEL:** __ **POST SUGAR LEVEL:** __								
LUNCH TOTALS								
SNACK / TIME: __								
DINNER / TIME: __ **INSULIN:** __ **PRE SUGAR LEVEL:** __ **POST SUGAR LEVEL:** __								
DINNER TOTALS								
SNACK / TIME: __								
DAILY TOTALS:								

VITAMINS / SUPPLEMENTS:
_____

EXERCISE:
_____

NOTES:
_____

DAILY BLOOD SUGAR LOG

DAY/DATE: _____

WEIGHT: _____

MOOD/ENERGY: _____

	Glycemic index	Glycemic load	Calories (kcal)	Carbs (g)	Fiber (g)	Total sugar (g)	Added sugar (g)	Protein (g)
BREAKFAST / TIME: ___ **INSULIN:** ___ **PRE SUGAR LEVEL:** ___ **POST SUGAR LEVEL:** ___								
BREAKFAST TOTALS								
SNACK / TIME: ___								
LUNCH / TIME: ___ **INSULIN:** ___ **PRE SUGAR LEVEL:** ___ **POST SUGAR LEVEL:** ___								
LUNCH TOTALS								
SNACK / TIME: ___								
DINNER / TIME: ___ **INSULIN:** ___ **PRE SUGAR LEVEL:** ___ **POST SUGAR LEVEL:** ___								
DINNER TOTALS								
SNACK / TIME: ___								
DAILY TOTALS:								

VITAMINS / SUPPLEMENTS:

EXERCISE:

NOTES:

DAILY BLOOD SUGAR LOG

DAY/DATE: _____

WEIGHT: _____

MOOD/ENERGY: _____

	Glycemic index	Glycemic load	Calories (kcal)	Carbs (g)	Fiber (g)	Total sugar (g)	Added sugar (g)	Protein (g)
BREAKFAST / TIME: ___ **INSULIN:** ___ **PRE SUGAR LEVEL:** ___ **POST SUGAR LEVEL:** ___								
BREAKFAST TOTALS								
SNACK / TIME:								
LUNCH / TIME: ___ **INSULIN:** ___ **PRE SUGAR LEVEL:** ___ **POST SUGAR LEVEL:** ___								
LUNCH TOTALS								
SNACK / TIME:								
DINNER / TIME: ___ **INSULIN:** ___ **PRE SUGAR LEVEL:** ___ **POST SUGAR LEVEL:** ___								
DINNER TOTALS								
SNACK / TIME:								
DAILY TOTALS:								

VITAMINS / SUPPLEMENTS:

EXERCISE:

NOTES:

DAILY BLOOD SUGAR LOG

DAY/DATE: _____

WEIGHT: _____

MOOD/ENERGY: _____

	Glycemic index	Glycemic load	Calories (kcal)	Carbs (g)	Fiber (g)	Total sugar (g)	Added sugar (g)	Protein (g)
BREAKFAST / TIME: [ ] **INSULIN:** [ ] **PRE SUGAR LEVEL:** [ ] **POST SUGAR LEVEL:** [ ]								
BREAKFAST TOTALS								
SNACK / TIME: [ ]								
LUNCH / TIME: [ ] **INSULIN:** [ ] **PRE SUGAR LEVEL:** [ ] **POST SUGAR LEVEL:** [ ]								
LUNCH TOTALS								
SNACK / TIME: [ ]								
DINNER / TIME: [ ] **INSULIN:** [ ] **PRE SUGAR LEVEL:** [ ] **POST SUGAR LEVEL:** [ ]								
DINNER TOTALS								
SNACK / TIME: [ ]								
DAILY TOTALS:								

VITAMINS / SUPPLEMENTS:

EXERCISE:

NOTES:

DAILY BLOOD SUGAR LOG

DAY/DATE: _____

WEIGHT: _____

MOOD/ENERGY: _____

	Glycemic index	Glycemic load	Calories (kcal)	Carbs (g)	Fiber (g)	Total sugar (g)	Added sugar (g)	Protein (g)
BREAKFAST / TIME: **INSULIN:** **PRE SUGAR LEVEL:** **POST SUGAR LEVEL:**								
BREAKFAST TOTALS								
SNACK / TIME:								
LUNCH / TIME: **INSULIN:** **PRE SUGAR LEVEL:** **POST SUGAR LEVEL:**								
LUNCH TOTALS								
SNACK / TIME:								
DINNER / TIME: **INSULIN:** **PRE SUGAR LEVEL:** **POST SUGAR LEVEL:**								
DINNER TOTALS								
SNACK / TIME:								
DAILY TOTALS:								

VITAMINS / SUPPLEMENTS:
_____

EXERCISE:
_____

NOTES:
_____

DAILY BLOOD SUGAR LOG

DAY / DATE: _____

WEIGHT: _____

MOOD / ENERGY: _____

	Glycemic index	Glycemic load	Calories (kcal)	Carbs (g)	Fiber (g)	Total sugar (g)	Added sugar (g)	Protein (g)
BREAKFAST / TIME: **INSULIN:** **PRE SUGAR LEVEL:** **POST SUGAR LEVEL:**								
BREAKFAST TOTALS								
SNACK / TIME:								
LUNCH / TIME: **INSULIN:** **PRE SUGAR LEVEL:** **POST SUGAR LEVEL:**								
LUNCH TOTALS								
SNACK / TIME:								
DINNER / TIME: **INSULIN:** **PRE SUGAR LEVEL:** **POST SUGAR LEVEL:**								
DINNER TOTALS								
SNACK / TIME:								
DAILY TOTALS:								

VITAMINS / SUPPLEMENTS:
_____

EXERCISE:
_____

NOTES:
_____

DAILY BLOOD SUGAR LOG

DAY/DATE: _____

WEIGHT: _____

MOOD/ENERGY: _____

	Glycemic index	Glycemic load	Calories (kcal)	Carbs (g)	Fiber (g)	Total sugar (g)	Added sugar (g)	Protein (g)
BREAKFAST / TIME: **INSULIN:** **PRE SUGAR LEVEL:** **POST SUGAR LEVEL:**								
BREAKFAST TOTALS								
SNACK / TIME:								
LUNCH / TIME: **INSULIN:** **PRE SUGAR LEVEL:** **POST SUGAR LEVEL:**								
LUNCH TOTALS								
SNACK / TIME:								
DINNER / TIME: **INSULIN:** **PRE SUGAR LEVEL:** **POST SUGAR LEVEL:**								
DINNER TOTALS								
SNACK / TIME:								
DAILY TOTALS:								

VITAMINS / SUPPLEMENTS: _____

EXERCISE: _____

NOTES: _____

DAILY BLOOD SUGAR LOG

DAY/DATE: _____

WEIGHT: _____

MOOD/ENERGY: _____

	Glycemic index	Glycemic load	Calories (kcal)	Carbs (g)	Fiber (g)	Total sugar (g)	Added sugar (g)	Protein (g)
BREAKFAST / TIME: — **INSULIN:** — **PRE SUGAR LEVEL:** — **POST SUGAR LEVEL:**								
BREAKFAST TOTALS								
SNACK / TIME:								
LUNCH / TIME: — **INSULIN:** — **PRE SUGAR LEVEL:** — **POST SUGAR LEVEL:**								
LUNCH TOTALS								
SNACK / TIME:								
DINNER / TIME: — **INSULIN:** — **PRE SUGAR LEVEL:** — **POST SUGAR LEVEL:**								
DINNER TOTALS								
SNACK / TIME:								
DAILY TOTALS:								

VITAMINS / SUPPLEMENTS:

_____

EXERCISE:

_____

NOTES:

_____

DAILY BLOOD SUGAR LOG

DAY/DATE: _____

WEIGHT: _____

MOOD/ENERGY: _____

	Glycemic index	Glycemic load	Calories (kcal)	Carbs (g)	Fiber (g)	Total sugar (g)	Added sugar (g)	Protein (g)
BREAKFAST / TIME: INSULIN: PRE SUGAR LEVEL: POST SUGAR LEVEL:								
BREAKFAST TOTALS								
SNACK / TIME:								
LUNCH / TIME: INSULIN: PRE SUGAR LEVEL: POST SUGAR LEVEL:								
LUNCH TOTALS								
SNACK / TIME:								
DINNER / TIME: INSULIN: PRE SUGAR LEVEL: POST SUGAR LEVEL:								
DINNER TOTALS								
SNACK / TIME:								
DAILY TOTALS:								

VITAMINS / SUPPLEMENTS:

EXERCISE:

NOTES:

DAILY BLOOD SUGAR LOG

DAY/DATE: _____

WEIGHT: _____

MOOD/ENERGY: _____

	Glycemic index	Glycemic load	Calories (kcal)	Carbs (g)	Fiber (g)	Total sugar (g)	Added sugar (g)	Protein (g)
BREAKFAST / TIME: INSULIN: PRE SUGAR LEVEL: POST SUGAR LEVEL:								
BREAKFAST TOTALS								
SNACK / TIME:								
LUNCH / TIME: INSULIN: PRE SUGAR LEVEL: POST SUGAR LEVEL:								
LUNCH TOTALS								
SNACK / TIME:								
DINNER / TIME: INSULIN: PRE SUGAR LEVEL: POST SUGAR LEVEL:								
DINNER TOTALS								
SNACK / TIME:								
DAILY TOTALS:								

VITAMINS / SUPPLEMENTS:

EXERCISE:

NOTES:

DAILY BLOOD SUGAR LOG

DAY/DATE: _____

WEIGHT: _____

MOOD/ENERGY: _____

	Glycemic index	Glycemic load	Calories (Kcal)	Carbs (g)	Fiber (g)	Total sugar (g)	Added sugar (g)	Protein (g)
BREAKFAST / TIME: INSULIN: PRE SUGAR LEVEL: POST SUGAR LEVEL:								
BREAKFAST TOTALS								
SNACK / TIME:								
LUNCH / TIME: INSULIN: PRE SUGAR LEVEL: POST SUGAR LEVEL:								
LUNCH TOTALS								
SNACK / TIME:								
DINNER / TIME: INSULIN: PRE SUGAR LEVEL: POST SUGAR LEVEL:								
DINNER TOTALS								
SNACK / TIME:								
DAILY TOTALS:								

VITAMINS / SUPPLEMENTS:
_____

EXERCISE:
_____

NOTES:
_____

DAILY BLOOD SUGAR LOG

DAY/DATE: _____

WEIGHT: _____

MOOD/ENERGY: _____

	Glycemic index	Glycemic load	Calories (kcal)	Carbs (g)	Fiber (g)	Total sugar (g)	Added sugar (g)	Protein (g)
BREAKFAST / TIME: ___ **INSULIN:** ___ **PRE SUGAR LEVEL:** ___ **POST SUGAR LEVEL:** ___								
BREAKFAST TOTALS								
SNACK / TIME: ___								
LUNCH / TIME: ___ **INSULIN:** ___ **PRE SUGAR LEVEL:** ___ **POST SUGAR LEVEL:** ___								
LUNCH TOTALS								
SNACK / TIME: ___								
DINNER / TIME: ___ **INSULIN:** ___ **PRE SUGAR LEVEL:** ___ **POST SUGAR LEVEL:** ___								
DINNER TOTALS								
SNACK / TIME: ___								
DAILY TOTALS:								

VITAMINS / SUPPLEMENTS:

EXERCISE:

NOTES:

DAILY BLOOD SUGAR LOG

DAY/DATE: _____

WEIGHT: _____

MOOD/ENERGY: _____

	Glycemic index	Glycemic load	Calories (kcal)	Carbs (g)	Fiber (g)	Total sugar (g)	Added sugar (g)	Protein (g)
BREAKFAST / TIME: **INSULIN:** **PRE SUGAR LEVEL:** **POST SUGAR LEVEL:**								
BREAKFAST TOTALS								
SNACK / TIME:								
LUNCH / TIME: **INSULIN:** **PRE SUGAR LEVEL:** **POST SUGAR LEVEL:**								
LUNCH TOTALS								
SNACK / TIME:								
DINNER / TIME: **INSULIN:** **PRE SUGAR LEVEL:** **POST SUGAR LEVEL:**								
DINNER TOTALS								
SNACK / TIME:								
DAILY TOTALS:								

VITAMINS / SUPPLEMENTS:

_____

EXERCISE:

_____

NOTES:

_____

DAILY BLOOD SUGAR LOG

DAY/DATE: _____

WEIGHT: _____

MOOD/ENERGY: _____

	Glycemic index	Glycemic load	Calories (kcal)	Carbs (g)	Fiber (g)	Total sugar (g)	Added sugar (g)	Protein (g)
BREAKFAST / TIME: ___ **INSULIN:** ___ **PRE SUGAR LEVEL:** ___ **POST SUGAR LEVEL:** ___								
BREAKFAST TOTALS								
SNACK / TIME: ___								
LUNCH / TIME: ___ **INSULIN:** ___ **PRE SUGAR LEVEL:** ___ **POST SUGAR LEVEL:** ___								
LUNCH TOTALS								
SNACK / TIME: ___								
DINNER / TIME: ___ **INSULIN:** ___ **PRE SUGAR LEVEL:** ___ **POST SUGAR LEVEL:** ___								
DINNER TOTALS								
SNACK / TIME: ___								
DAILY TOTALS:								

VITAMINS / SUPPLEMENTS: _____

EXERCISE: _____

NOTES: _____

DAILY BLOOD SUGAR LOG

DAY/DATE: _____

WEIGHT: _____

MOOD/ENERGY: _____

	Glycemic index	Glycemic load	Calories (kcal)	Carbs (g)	Fiber (g)	Total sugar (g)	Added sugar (g)	Protein (g)
BREAKFAST / TIME: _____ **INSULIN:** _____ **PRE SUGAR LEVEL:** _____ **POST SUGAR LEVEL:** _____								
BREAKFAST TOTALS								
SNACK / TIME: _____								
LUNCH / TIME: _____ **INSULIN:** _____ **PRE SUGAR LEVEL:** _____ **POST SUGAR LEVEL:** _____								
LUNCH TOTALS								
SNACK / TIME: _____								
DINNER / TIME: _____ **INSULIN:** _____ **PRE SUGAR LEVEL:** _____ **POST SUGAR LEVEL:** _____								
DINNER TOTALS								
SNACK / TIME: _____								
DAILY TOTALS:								

VITAMINS / SUPPLEMENTS:
_____

EXERCISE:
_____

NOTES:
_____

DAILY BLOOD SUGAR LOG

DAY/DATE: _____

WEIGHT: _____

MOOD/ENERGY: _____

	Glycemic index	Glycemic load	Calories (kcal)	Carbs (g)	Fiber (g)	Total sugar (g)	Added sugar (g)	Protein (g)
BREAKFAST / TIME: INSULIN: PRE SUGAR LEVEL: POST SUGAR LEVEL:								
BREAKFAST TOTALS								
SNACK / TIME:								
LUNCH / TIME: INSULIN: PRE SUGAR LEVEL: POST SUGAR LEVEL:								
LUNCH TOTALS								
SNACK / TIME:								
DINNER / TIME: INSULIN: PRE SUGAR LEVEL: POST SUGAR LEVEL:								
DINNER TOTALS								
SNACK / TIME:								
DAILY TOTALS:								

VITAMINS / SUPPLEMENTS:

EXERCISE:

NOTES:

DAILY BLOOD SUGAR LOG

DAY/DATE: _____

WEIGHT: _____

MOOD/ENERGY: _____

	Glycemic index	Glycemic load	Calories (kcal)	Carbs (g)	Fiber (g)	Total sugar (g)	Added sugar (g)	Protein (g)
BREAKFAST / TIME: **INSULIN:** **PRE SUGAR LEVEL:** **POST SUGAR LEVEL:**								
BREAKFAST TOTALS								
SNACK / TIME:								
LUNCH / TIME: **INSULIN:** **PRE SUGAR LEVEL:** **POST SUGAR LEVEL:**								
LUNCH TOTALS								
SNACK / TIME:								
DINNER / TIME: **INSULIN:** **PRE SUGAR LEVEL:** **POST SUGAR LEVEL:**								
DINNER TOTALS								
SNACK / TIME:								
DAILY TOTALS:								

VITAMINS / SUPPLEMENTS:
_____

EXERCISE:
_____

NOTES:
_____

DAILY BLOOD SUGAR LOG

DAY/DATE: _____

WEIGHT: _____

MOOD/ENERGY: _____

	Glycemic index	Glycemic load	Calories (kcal)	Carbs (g)	Fiber (g)	Total sugar (g)	Added sugar (g)	Protein (g)
BREAKFAST / TIME: __ **INSULIN:** __ **PRE SUGAR LEVEL:** __ **POST SUGAR LEVEL:** __								
BREAKFAST TOTALS								
SNACK / TIME: __								
LUNCH / TIME: __ **INSULIN:** __ **PRE SUGAR LEVEL:** __ **POST SUGAR LEVEL:** __								
LUNCH TOTALS								
SNACK / TIME: __								
DINNER / TIME: __ **INSULIN:** __ **PRE SUGAR LEVEL:** __ **POST SUGAR LEVEL:** __								
DINNER TOTALS								
SNACK / TIME: __								
DAILY TOTALS:								

VITAMINS / SUPPLEMENTS:

EXERCISE:

NOTES:

DAILY BLOOD SUGAR LOG

DAY/DATE: _____

WEIGHT: _____

MOOD/ENERGY: _____

	Glycemic index	Glycemic load	Calories (kcal)	Carbs (g)	Fiber (g)	Total sugar (g)	Added sugar (g)	Protein (g)
BREAKFAST / TIME: **INSULIN:** **PRE SUGAR LEVEL:** **POST SUGAR LEVEL:**								
BREAKFAST TOTALS								
SNACK / TIME:								
LUNCH / TIME: **INSULIN:** **PRE SUGAR LEVEL:** **POST SUGAR LEVEL:**								
LUNCH TOTALS								
SNACK / TIME:								
DINNER / TIME: **INSULIN:** **PRE SUGAR LEVEL:** **POST SUGAR LEVEL:**								
DINNER TOTALS								
SNACK / TIME:								
DAILY TOTALS:								

VITAMINS / SUPPLEMENTS:

EXERCISE:

NOTES:

DAILY BLOOD SUGAR LOG

DAY/DATE: _____

WEIGHT: _____

MOOD/ENERGY: _____

	Glycemic index	Glycemic load	Calories (kcal)	Carbs (g)	Fiber (g)	Total sugar (g)	Added sugar (g)	Protein (g)
BREAKFAST / TIME: INSULIN: PRE SUGAR LEVEL: POST SUGAR LEVEL:								
BREAKFAST TOTALS								
SNACK / TIME:								
LUNCH / TIME: INSULIN: PRE SUGAR LEVEL: POST SUGAR LEVEL:								
LUNCH TOTALS								
SNACK / TIME:								
DINNER / TIME: INSULIN: PRE SUGAR LEVEL: POST SUGAR LEVEL:								
DINNER TOTALS								
SNACK / TIME:								
DAILY TOTALS:								

VITAMINS / SUPPLEMENTS:

EXERCISE:

NOTES:

DAILY BLOOD SUGAR LOG

DAY/DATE: _____

WEIGHT: _____

MOOD/ENERGY: _____

	Glycemic index	Glycemic load	Calories (kcal)	Carbs (g)	Fiber (g)	Total sugar (g)	Added sugar (g)	Protein (g)
BREAKFAST / TIME: INSULIN: PRE SUGAR LEVEL: POST SUGAR LEVEL:								
BREAKFAST TOTALS								
SNACK / TIME:								
LUNCH / TIME: INSULIN: PRE SUGAR LEVEL: POST SUGAR LEVEL:								
LUNCH TOTALS								
SNACK / TIME:								
DINNER / TIME: INSULIN: PRE SUGAR LEVEL: POST SUGAR LEVEL:								
DINNER TOTALS								
SNACK / TIME:								
DAILY TOTALS:								

VITAMINS / SUPPLEMENTS:
_____

EXERCISE:
_____

NOTES:
_____

DAILY BLOOD SUGAR LOG

DAY/DATE: _____

WEIGHT: _____

MOOD/ENERGY: _____

	Glycemic index	Glycemic load	Calories (kcal)	Carbs (g)	Fiber (g)	Total sugar (g)	Added sugar (g)	Protein (g)
BREAKFAST / TIME: ___ **INSULIN:** ___ **PRE SUGAR LEVEL:** ___ **POST SUGAR LEVEL:** ___								
BREAKFAST TOTALS								
SNACK / TIME: ___								
LUNCH / TIME: ___ **INSULIN:** ___ **PRE SUGAR LEVEL:** ___ **POST SUGAR LEVEL:** ___								
LUNCH TOTALS								
SNACK / TIME: ___								
DINNER / TIME: ___ **INSULIN:** ___ **PRE SUGAR LEVEL:** ___ **POST SUGAR LEVEL:** ___								
DINNER TOTALS								
SNACK / TIME: ___								
DAILY TOTALS:								

VITAMINS / SUPPLEMENTS:

EXERCISE:

NOTES:

DAILY BLOOD SUGAR LOG

DAY / DATE: _____

WEIGHT: _____

MOOD / ENERGY: _____

	Glycemic index	Glycemic load	Calories (kcal)	Carbs (g)	Fiber (g)	Total sugar (g)	Added sugar (g)	Protein (g)
BREAKFAST / TIME: ___ **INSULIN:** ___ **PRE SUGAR LEVEL:** ___ **POST SUGAR LEVEL:** ___								
BREAKFAST TOTALS								
SNACK / TIME: ___								
LUNCH / TIME: ___ **INSULIN:** ___ **PRE SUGAR LEVEL:** ___ **POST SUGAR LEVEL:** ___								
LUNCH TOTALS								
SNACK / TIME: ___								
DINNER / TIME: ___ **INSULIN:** ___ **PRE SUGAR LEVEL:** ___ **POST SUGAR LEVEL:** ___								
DINNER TOTALS								
SNACK / TIME: ___								
DAILY TOTALS:								

VITAMINS / SUPPLEMENTS:

_____

EXERCISE:

_____

_____

NOTES:

_____

DAILY BLOOD SUGAR LOG

DAY/DATE: _____

WEIGHT: _____

MOOD/ENERGY: _____

	Glycemic index	Glycemic load	Calories (kcal)	Carbs (g)	Fiber (g)	Total sugar (g)	Added sugar (g)	Protein (g)
BREAKFAST / TIME: **INSULIN:** **PRE SUGAR LEVEL:** **POST SUGAR LEVEL:**								
BREAKFAST TOTALS								
SNACK / TIME:								
LUNCH / TIME: **INSULIN:** **PRE SUGAR LEVEL:** **POST SUGAR LEVEL:**								
LUNCH TOTALS								
SNACK / TIME:								
DINNER / TIME: **INSULIN:** **PRE SUGAR LEVEL:** **POST SUGAR LEVEL:**								
DINNER TOTALS								
SNACK / TIME:								
DAILY TOTALS:								

VITAMINS / SUPPLEMENTS:

EXERCISE:

NOTES:

DAILY BLOOD SUGAR LOG

DAY/DATE: _____

WEIGHT: _____

MOOD/ENERGY: _____

	Glycemic index	Glycemic load	Calories (Kcal)	Carbs (g)	Fiber (g)	Total sugar (g)	Added sugar (g)	Protein (g)
BREAKFAST / TIME: ___ **INSULIN:** ___ **PRE SUGAR LEVEL:** ___ **POST SUGAR LEVEL:** ___								
BREAKFAST TOTALS								
SNACK / TIME: ___								
LUNCH / TIME: ___ **INSULIN:** ___ **PRE SUGAR LEVEL:** ___ **POST SUGAR LEVEL:** ___								
LUNCH TOTALS								
SNACK / TIME: ___								
DINNER / TIME: ___ **INSULIN:** ___ **PRE SUGAR LEVEL:** ___ **POST SUGAR LEVEL:** ___								
DINNER TOTALS								
SNACK / TIME: ___								
DAILY TOTALS:								

VITAMINS / SUPPLEMENTS:

EXERCISE:

NOTES:

DAILY BLOOD SUGAR LOG

DAY/DATE: _____

WEIGHT: _____

MOOD/ENERGY: _____

	Glycemic index	Glycemic load	Calories (kcal)	Carbs (g)	Fiber (g)	Total sugar (g)	Added sugar (g)	Protein (g)
BREAKFAST / TIME: INSULIN: PRE SUGAR LEVEL: POST SUGAR LEVEL:								
BREAKFAST TOTALS								
SNACK / TIME:								
LUNCH / TIME: INSULIN: PRE SUGAR LEVEL: POST SUGAR LEVEL:								
LUNCH TOTALS								
SNACK / TIME:								
DINNER / TIME: INSULIN: PRE SUGAR LEVEL: POST SUGAR LEVEL:								
DINNER TOTALS								
SNACK / TIME:								
DAILY TOTALS:								

VITAMINS / SUPPLEMENTS: _____

EXERCISE: _____

NOTES: _____

DAILY BLOOD SUGAR LOG

DAY / DATE: _____

WEIGHT: _____

MOOD / ENERGY: _____

	Glycemic index	Glycemic load	Calories (kcal)	Carbs (g)	Fiber (g)	Total sugar (g)	Added sugar (g)	Protein (g)
BREAKFAST / TIME: **INSULIN:** **PRE SUGAR LEVEL:** **POST SUGAR LEVEL:**								
BREAKFAST TOTALS								
SNACK / TIME:								
LUNCH / TIME: **INSULIN:** **PRE SUGAR LEVEL:** **POST SUGAR LEVEL:**								
LUNCH TOTALS								
SNACK / TIME:								
DINNER / TIME: **INSULIN:** **PRE SUGAR LEVEL:** **POST SUGAR LEVEL:**								
DINNER TOTALS								
SNACK / TIME:								
DAILY TOTALS:								

VITAMINS / SUPPLEMENTS:
_____

EXERCISE:
_____

NOTES:
_____

DAILY BLOOD SUGAR LOG

DAY/DATE: _____

WEIGHT: _____

MOOD/ENERGY: _____

	Glycemic index	Glycemic load	Calories (kcal)	Carbs (g)	Fiber (g)	Total sugar (g)	Added sugar (g)	Protein (g)
BREAKFAST / TIME: ___ **INSULIN:** ___ **PRE SUGAR LEVEL:** ___ **POST SUGAR LEVEL:** ___								
BREAKFAST TOTALS								
SNACK / TIME:								
LUNCH / TIME: ___ **INSULIN:** ___ **PRE SUGAR LEVEL:** ___ **POST SUGAR LEVEL:** ___								
LUNCH TOTALS								
SNACK / TIME:								
DINNER / TIME: ___ **INSULIN:** ___ **PRE SUGAR LEVEL:** ___ **POST SUGAR LEVEL:** ___								
DINNER TOTALS								
SNACK / TIME:								
DAILY TOTALS:								

VITAMINS / SUPPLEMENTS:

EXERCISE:

NOTES:

DAILY BLOOD SUGAR LOG

DAY / DATE: _____

WEIGHT: _____

MOOD / ENERGY: _____

	Glycemic index	Glycemic load	Calories (kcal)	Carbs (g)	Fiber (g)	Total sugar (g)	Added sugar (g)	Protein (g)
BREAKFAST / TIME: INSULIN: PRE SUGAR LEVEL: POST SUGAR LEVEL:								
BREAKFAST TOTALS								
SNACK / TIME:								
LUNCH / TIME: INSULIN: PRE SUGAR LEVEL: POST SUGAR LEVEL:								
LUNCH TOTALS								
SNACK / TIME:								
DINNER / TIME: INSULIN: PRE SUGAR LEVEL: POST SUGAR LEVEL:								
DINNER TOTALS								
SNACK / TIME:								
DAILY TOTALS:								

VITAMINS / SUPPLEMENTS:

EXERCISE:

NOTES:

DAILY BLOOD SUGAR LOG

DAY/DATE: _____

WEIGHT: _____

MOOD/ENERGY: _____

	Glycemic index	Glycemic load	Calories (kcal)	Carbs (g)	Fiber (g)	Total sugar (g)	Added sugar (g)	Protein (g)
BREAKFAST / TIME: INSULIN: PRE SUGAR LEVEL: POST SUGAR LEVEL:								
BREAKFAST TOTALS								
SNACK / TIME:								
LUNCH / TIME: INSULIN: PRE SUGAR LEVEL: POST SUGAR LEVEL:								
LUNCH TOTALS								
SNACK / TIME:								
DINNER / TIME: INSULIN: PRE SUGAR LEVEL: POST SUGAR LEVEL:								
DINNER TOTALS								
SNACK / TIME:								
DAILY TOTALS:								

VITAMINS / SUPPLEMENTS:

EXERCISE:

NOTES:

DAILY BLOOD SUGAR LOG

DAY/DATE: _____

WEIGHT: _____

MOOD/ENERGY: _____

	Glycemic index	Glycemic load	Calories (kcal)	Carbs (g)	Fiber (g)	Total sugar (g)	Added sugar (g)	Protein (g)
BREAKFAST / TIME: **INSULIN:** **PRE SUGAR LEVEL:** **POST SUGAR LEVEL:**								
BREAKFAST TOTALS								
SNACK / TIME:								
LUNCH / TIME: **INSULIN:** **PRE SUGAR LEVEL:** **POST SUGAR LEVEL:**								
LUNCH TOTALS								
SNACK / TIME:								
DINNER / TIME: **INSULIN:** **PRE SUGAR LEVEL:** **POST SUGAR LEVEL:**								
DINNER TOTALS								
SNACK / TIME:								
DAILY TOTALS:								

VITAMINS / SUPPLEMENTS:
_____

EXERCISE:
_____

NOTES:
_____

DAILY BLOOD SUGAR LOG

DAY/DATE: _____

WEIGHT: _____

MOOD/ENERGY: _____

	Glycemic index	Glycemic load	Calories (kcal)	Carbs (g)	Fiber (g)	Total sugar (g)	Added sugar (g)	Protein (g)
BREAKFAST / TIME:	**INSULIN:**		**PRE SUGAR LEVEL:**			**POST SUGAR LEVEL:**		
BREAKFAST TOTALS								
SNACK / TIME:								
LUNCH / TIME:	**INSULIN:**		**PRE SUGAR LEVEL:**			**POST SUGAR LEVEL:**		
LUNCH TOTALS								
SNACK / TIME:								
DINNER / TIME:	**INSULIN:**		**PRE SUGAR LEVEL:**			**POST SUGAR LEVEL:**		
DINNER TOTALS								
SNACK / TIME:								
DAILY TOTALS:								

VITAMINS / SUPPLEMENTS:

EXERCISE:

NOTES:

DAILY BLOOD SUGAR LOG

DAY/DATE: _____

WEIGHT: _____

MOOD/ENERGY: _____

	Glycemic index	Glycemic load	Calories (kcal)	Carbs (g)	Fiber (g)	Total sugar (g)	Added sugar (g)	Protein (g)
BREAKFAST / TIME: INSULIN: PRE SUGAR LEVEL: POST SUGAR LEVEL:								
BREAKFAST TOTALS								
SNACK / TIME:								
LUNCH / TIME: INSULIN: PRE SUGAR LEVEL: POST SUGAR LEVEL:								
LUNCH TOTALS								
SNACK / TIME:								
DINNER / TIME: INSULIN: PRE SUGAR LEVEL: POST SUGAR LEVEL:								
DINNER TOTALS								
SNACK / TIME:								
DAILY TOTALS:								

VITAMINS / SUPPLEMENTS:

EXERCISE:

NOTES:

NUTRITIONAL FACTS FOR POPULAR FOODS

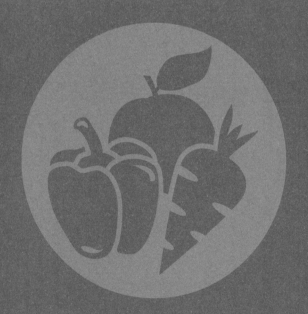

*Let food be your medicine
and medicine be your food*
—HIPPOCRATES

The following compilation of nutritional information of common foods is a handy reference for those tracking calories, fats, carbs, fiber, sugars, and protein, and being mindful of the glycemic index (GI) and glycemic load (GL).

F oods that have no discernible carbohydrate—meats, fish, chicken, tofu, nuts, eggs, avocados, many fruits and vegetables, wine, beer, and spirits—also have no glycemic index ranking, and so are not included in this list.

A disclaimer about the variability of the glycemic index and glycemic load:
The GI values, generated and compiled by Sydney University's Glycemic Index Research Service, represents high-quality data from many studies done around the world. However, because the GI and GL numbers were calculated in different experiments through different organizations in different countries, there might be variations in how the item was made or cooked. The GI of some processed foods may vary in different places and times due to differences in manufacturing, and the GI of some produce may vary depending on differences in where and how each food was raised. Some foods' GI may even differ depending on the testing methods used to determine their index numbers.

That said, the source data our editors have used to compile the following pages is the most accurate to date. The editors have done their best to select entries that are the most common worldwide and that are subject to the least ambiguity. Readers may also find that amounts of foods do not always reflect a normal or appropriate serving size; this is a reflection of the amounts used in reference studies.

Although the charts contained on the following pages may be handy, please note that they are for general informational purposes only and should not be taken as a substitute for advice from a medical practitioner. As always, consult your physician before making any decision concerning your diet.

Furthermore, the nutrient values of prepared foods are subject to change and may differ from the listings in this book. Nutrient values for calories, fats, carbs, fiber, sugar, and protein are based on USDA guidelines. The reference source for glycemic index and glycemic load data is the International Tables of Glycemic Index and Glycemic Load Values: 2008, copyright © 2008 the Institute of Obesity, Nutrition and Exercise, University of Sydney, New South Wales, Australia. Used by permission.

Description of food	Glycemic index	Glycemic load (per serving)	Calories (kcal)
AGAVE cactus nectar, high-fructose, 10g (0.4oz)	13	1	33
APPLE, dried, 60g (2.1oz)	29±5	11	146
APPLE, golden delicious, 120g (4.2oz)	39±3	6	62
APPLE JUICE, unsweetened, 250mL (1.1cup)	44±2	13	123
APRICOT, 100% pure fruit spread, 30g (1.1oz)	43±6	7	75
APRICOTS, canned in fruit juice, 120g (4.2oz)	51±5	6	58
APRICOTS, dried, 60g (2.1oz)	31	7	145
APRICOTS, fresh, 120g (4.2oz)	34±3	3	58
BAKED BEANS, canned, 150g (5.3oz)	40±3	6	141
BANANA, 120g (4.2oz)	62±9	16	107
BARLEY, cooked, 150g (5.3oz)	28±2	12	183
BEER, 250mL (1.1cup)	66±7	5	109
BLACK BEANS, boiled, 150g (5.3oz)	20	5	198
BLACKBERRY, 100% fruit spread, 30g (1.1oz)	46±5	8	58
BLACKEYED PEAS, boiled, 150g (5.3oz)	33±4	10	174
BLUEBERRIES, wild, 100g (3.5oz)	53±7	5	57
BREAD, bagel, white, 70g (2.5oz)	69	24	180
BREAD, baguette, 30g (1.1oz)	57±9	10	82
BREAD, English muffin, 30g (1.1oz)	77±7	11	68
BREAD, English muffin, multigrain, 30g (1.1oz)	45±3	5	70
BREAD, Healthy Choice Hearty 7-Grain, 30g (1.1oz)	55±6	8	64
BREAD, Healthy Choice whole grain, 30g (1.1oz)	62±6	9	70
BREAD, oat, 30g (1.1oz)	65	12	71
BREAD, pita, white, 30g (1.1oz)	68±5	10	82
BREAD, pita, wholemeal, 30g (1.1oz)	56±13	8	80
BREAD, roll, whole wheat burger, 30g (1.1oz)	62±6	7	84
BREAD, roll, whole wheat hot dog, 30g (1.1oz)	62±6	7	66
BREAD, rye, 30g (1.1oz)	50	7	78

Fat (grams)	Carbs (grams)	Fiber (grams)	Sugar (grams)	Protein (grams)
0	8	1	7	0
0	40	5	34	1
0	17	3	13	0
0	31	0	29	0
0	20	0	20	0
0	15	2	13	1
0	38	4	32	2
1	13	2	11	2
1	32	6	12	7
0	27	3	15	1
1	42	6	0	3
0	9	0	0	1
0	36	13	0	13
0	13	0	13	0
1	31	10	5	12
0	15	2	10	1
1	35	2	4	7
1	16	1	0	3
1	13	1	1	3
1	14	1	0	3
1	14	2	2	3
1	13	4	3	4
1	12	1	2	3
0	17	1	0	3
1	17	2	0	3
2	13	2	3	4
1	13	2	1	3
1	15	2	1	3

Description of food	Glycemic index	Glycemic load (per serving)	Calories (kcal)
BREAD, white, 30g (1.1oz)	75±2	11	80
BREAD, whole wheat, 30g (1.1oz)	74±2	9	78
BREAD, Wonder enriched white, 30g (1.1oz)	71	10	74
CAKE, banana, 60g (2.1oz)	47±8	14	179
CAKE, chocolate, from mix, frosted, 111g (3.9oz)	38±3	20	432
CAKE, vanilla, from mix, frosted, 111g (3.9oz)	42±4	24	414
CANDY, chocolate, dark, Dove 50g (1.8oz)	23±3	6	260
CANDY, chocolate, milk, 50g (1.8oz)	43±3	12	268
CANDY, jelly beans, 30g (1.1oz)	80±8	22	120
CANDY, licorice, soft, 30g (1.1oz)	78±11	16	112
CANDY, M&M's, peanut, 30g (1.1oz)	33±3	6	154
CANDY, Mars Bar, 60g (2.1oz)	68±12	27	280
CANDY, Milky Way bar, 60g (2.1oz)	62	26	274
CANDY, Skittles, 50g (1.8oz)	70±5	32	202
CANDY, Snickers bar, 60g (2.1oz)	51	18	295
CANDY, Twix cookie bar, 60g (2.1oz)	44	17	301
CANTALOUPE, fresh, 120g (4.2oz)	65±9	4	41
CARROT JUICE, fresh, 250mL (1.1cup)	43±3	10	100
CARROTS, 80g (2.8oz)	39±4	2	33
CEREAL, All-Bran (Kellogg's), 30g (1.1oz)	44±6	9	78
CEREAL, Corn Pops (Kellogg's), 30g (1.1oz)	80	21	120
CEREAL, cornflakes, 30g (1.1oz)	81±3	20	108
CEREAL, Froot Loops (Kellogg's), 30g (1.1oz)	69±9	18	112
CEREAL, Grape-nuts (Kraft), 30g (1.1oz)	67	13	108
CEREAL, Just Right (Kellogg's), 30g (1.1oz)	60±15	13	117
CEREAL, Kashi Seven Whole Grain Puffs, 30g (1.1oz)	65	16	100

Fat (grams)	Carbs (grams)	Fiber (grams)	Sugar (grams)	Protein (grams)
1	15	1	1	2
1	14	1	2	3
1	15	1	3	2
4	34	1	24	2
22	59	2	44	4
16	65	0	40	4
16	30	4	23	3
15	30	2	26	4
0	30	0	30	0
0	28	0	21	0
8	18	1	15	3
14	38	1	31	5
10	43	1	36	2
2	45	0	38	0
14	37	1	30	5
15	39	1	29	3
0	10	1	9	1
0	23	2	10	2
0	8	2	4	1
1	22	9	5	4
0	27	3	9	1
0	26	1	2	2
1	26	3	13	2
1	24	4	3	3
1	24	2	5	3
1	22	3	0	4

Description of food	Glycemic index	Glycemic load (per serving)	Calories (kcal)
CEREAL, Mini-Wheats (Kellogg's), 30g (1.1oz)	58±8	12	104
CEREAL, muesli (Alpen), 30g (1.1oz)	55±10	11	116
CEREAL, Raisin Bran (Kellogg's), 30g (1.1oz)	61±5	12	95
CEREAL, Special K, 30g (1.1oz)	69±5	14	113
CEREAL, Weetabix, 30g (1.1oz)	75	16	111
CHERRIES, dark, pitted, 120g (4.2oz)	63±6	9	75
CHICKPEAS, boiled, 150g (5.3oz)	36±5	11	246
COOKIES, arrowroot, 25g (0.9oz)	69±7	12	108
COOKIES, digestives, 25g (0.9oz)	59±7	9	125
COOKIES, macaroons, 30g (1.1oz)	32	6	117
COOKIES, oatmeal, 25g (0.9oz)	54±4	9	112
COOKIES, Rich Tea biscuits, 25g (0.9oz)	55±4	10	113
CORN, sweet, cooked, 150g (5.3oz)	52±5	17	144
CORN CHIPS, Doritos, 50g (1.8oz)	72	18	249
COUSCOUS, cooked, 150g (5.3oz)	65±7	9	168
CRACKER, water, 25g (0.9oz)	63±9	11	126
CRACKER, RICE, plain, 30g (1.1oz)	91	23	115
CRANBERRY JUICE COCKTAIL, 250mL (1.1cup)	59	19	144
CUSTARD, homemade from milk, 100g (3.5oz)	43±10	7	95
DATES, dried, 60g (2.1oz)	42±4	18	169
DOUGHNUT, wheat, 50g (1.8oz)	75±7	15	180
ENERGY BAR, Clif chocolate brownie, 65g (2.3oz)	57	22	250
ENERGY BAR, Power Bar Performance chocolate, 65g (2.3oz)	58	24	220
ENSURE pudding, vanilla, 113g (4oz)	36±4	9	147
ENSURE vanilla drink, 237mL (1 cup)	50	19	220
FIGS, dried, 60g (2.1oz)	61±6	16	149
FROZEN YOGURT, 125g (4.4oz)	51	11	134
FRUIT, mixed dried, 60g (2.1oz)	60±7	24	146
FRUIT DRINK, punch, 250mL (1.1cup)	67	19	120

Fat (grams)	Carbs (grams)	Fiber (grams)	Sugar (grams)	Protein (grams)
1	26	3	7	3
2	22	3	4	4
0	23	3	9	3
1	22	0	4	6
1	24	3	2	3
0	19	3	15	1
4	41	11	7	13
3	19	2	8	2
5	17	1	4	2
6	17	1	8	1
5	17	1	6	2
4	19	1	5	2
2	31	4	7	5
13	32	2	0	4
0	35	2	0	6
6	15	0	1	2
2	22	1	0	2
0	36	0	32	0
4	11	0	11	5
0	45	5	38	2
10	21	1	11	3
5	45	5	22	9
3	45	3	26	9
4	25	0	23	3
6	32	0	15	9
1	38	6	29	2
2	25	0	24	6
0	38	5	29	2
0	31	0	28	0

Description of food	Glycemic index	Glycemic load (per serving)	Calories (kcal)
FRUIT DRINK, smoothie, soy & banana, 250mL (1.1cup)	30±3	7	210
FRUIT DRINK, V8 Splash Smoothie, banana & strawberry, 250mL (1.1cup)	44±3	11	94
FRUIT DRINK, V8 Splash, tropical blend fruit drink, 250mL (1.1cup)	47±4	13	73
FRUIT SALAD, canned in juice, 120g (4.2oz)	54±3	6	60
GATORADE, 250mL (1.1cup)	78±13	12	56
GNOCCHI, 180g (6.3oz)	68±9	33	360
GRAPEFRUIT, ruby red, canned in juice, 120g (4.2oz)	47±5	10	44
GRAPES, black, 120g (4.2oz)	59	11	83
HONEY, 25g (0.9oz)	61±3	12	76
HOT CHOCOLATE, from mix with water, 250mL (1.1cup)	51±3	12	159
HUMMUS, 30g (1.1oz)	6±4	0	53
ICE CREAM, half vanilla, half chocolate, 50g (1.8oz)	57	6	94
ICE CREAM, low fat light, vanilla, 50g (1.8oz)	46	7	82
ICE CREAM, premium chocolate, 15% fat, 50g (1.8oz)	37±3	4	128
KIDNEY BEANS, boiled, 150g (5.3oz)	22±3	6	190
KIWI, 120g (4.2oz)	58±7	7	73
LENTILS, boiled, 150g (5.3oz)	29±3	5	174
LIMA BEANS, boiled, 150g (5.3oz)	32±3	7	170
LYCHEE, canned in syrup & drained, 120g (4.2oz)	79±8	16	109
MANGO, 120g (4.2oz)	51±3	8	78
MARSHMALLOWS, 30g (1.1oz)	62±6	15	95
MILK, condensed, sweetened, 100g (3.5oz)	61±6	33	321
MILK, low fat chocolate (made with Quik mix), 250mL (1.1cup)	41±4	5	167
MILK, reduced fat, 250mL (1.1cup)	30	4	129
MILK, skim, 250mL (1.1cup)	31±2	4	91
MILK, whole, 250mL (1.1cup)	31±4	4	155

Fat (grams)	Carbs (grams)	Fiber (grams)	Sugar (grams)	Protein (grams)
3	44	3	36	4
0	21	0	19	3
0	19	0	17	0
0	16	1	13	1
0	15	0	15	0
2	79	9	2	9
0	11	1	11	1
0	22	1	19	1
0	21	0	21	0
2	33	1	26	3
3	6	1	0	2
5	11	0	9	1
2	13	0	11	2
8	10	0	9	2
1	34	10	1	13
1	18	4	11	1
1	30	12	3	14
1	30	11	4	12
0	28	1	27	1
0	20	2	18	1
0	24	0	17	1
9	54	0	54	8
4	26	1	25	8
5	12	0	13	9
1	13	0	13	9
8	12	0	14	8

Description of food	Glycemic index	Glycemic load (per serving)	Calories (kcal)
MUFFIN, apple & oats, 60g (2.1oz)	44±6	13	175
MUFFIN, blueberry, Sara Lee, 60g (2.1oz)	50±3	15	180
NAVY BEANS, boiled, 150g (5.3oz)	31±6	9	210
NECTARINES, 120g (4.2oz)	43±6	4	53
NUTELLA chocolate hazelnut spread, 20g (0.7oz)	29	3	111
NUTS, cashew, roasted, 50g (1.8oz)	25±1	3	287
NUTS, mixed, roasted, 50g (1.8oz)	24±10	4	308
OATMEAL (instant porridge), 250g (8.8oz)	79±3	21	228
OATMEAL (porridge), 250g (8.8oz)	55±2	13	155
ORANGE, 120g (4.2oz)	40±3	4	56
ORANGE, mandarin segments, canned in juice, 120g (4.2oz)	47±2	6	44
ORANGE JUICE, 250mL (1.1cup)	50±2	12	118
ORANGE MARMALADE, 30g (1.1oz)	43	8	74
PANCAKES, homemade, 80g (2.8oz)	66±9	17	182
PANCAKES, wheat, 80g (2.8oz)	80±4	16	183
PASTA, fusilli twists, 180g (6.3oz)	55±2	25	240
PASTA, linguine, 180g (6.3oz)	52±3	23	284
PASTA, rice noodles, 180g (6.3oz)	61±6	23	196
PASTA, spaghetti, 180g (6.3oz)	49±3	24	284
PASTA, spaghetti, wholemeal, 180g (6.3oz)	42±4	17	221
PEACHES, canned in juice, 120g (4.2oz)	40	5	53
PEACHES, dried, 60g (2.1oz)	35±5	8	143
PEARS, canned in juice, 120g (4.2oz)	43±15	5	60
PINEAPPLE, canned in juice, 120g (4.2oz)	43±4	8	72
PINEAPPLE, fresh, 120g (4.2oz)	66±7	6	58
PINTO BEANS, boiled, 150g (5.3oz)	14	4	214
POPCORN, 20g (0.7oz)	65±5	7	108
POTATO, baked, 150g (5.3oz)	86±6	22	141
POTATO, boiled, 150g (5.3oz)	82±7	21	130
POTATO, French fries, Ore-Ida, 150g (5.3oz)	64±6	21	229

Fat (grams)	Carbs (grams)	Fiber (grams)	Sugar (grams)	Protein (grams)
6	29	3	6	4
5	31	1	14	2
1	39	16	1	12
0	13	2	10	1
6	12	1	12	2
23	16	2	3	8
28	11	3	2	8
3	46	5	17	6
3	27	4	1	7
0	14	3	11	1
0	12	1	11	1
1	27	1	22	2
0	20	0	18	0
8	23	0	0	5
8	23	3	5	6
1	50	2	2	8
2	56	3	1	10
0	45	2	0	2
2	56	3	1	10
1	48	8	1	10
0	14	2	12	1
1	37	5	25	2
0	16	2	12	0
0	19	2	17	1
0	15	2	11	1
1	39	14	1	14
7	12	2	0	2
0	32	3	2	3
0	30	3	1	3
8	35	4	2	4

Description of food	Glycemic index	Glycemic load (per serving)	Calories (kcal)
POTATO, instant mashed, 150g (5.3oz)	87±3	17	144
POTATO, instant mashed with 37g butter, 150g (5.3oz)	74±10	18	146
POTATO, mashed, 150g (5.3oz)	76	15	150
POTATO CHIPS, 50g (1.8oz)	56	12	274
PRETZELS, 30g (1.1oz)	84±6	20	114
PRUNE JUICE, 250mL (1.1cup)	43±3	15	192
PRUNES, pitted, 60g (2.1oz)	29±4	10	150
PUDDING, chocolate mix made with whole milk, 100g (3.5oz)	47±4	7	119
PUDDING, vanilla mix made with whole milk, 100g (3.5oz)	40±4	6	112
PUMPKIN, boiled, 80g (2.8oz)	64	6	21
PURE-PROTEIN BAR, chocolate, 80g (2.8oz)	38±4	5	288
PURE-PROTEIN BAR, peanut butter, 80g (2.8oz)	22±4	2	309
QUINOA, cooked, 150g (5.3oz)	53±5	13	214
RAISINS, 60g (2.1oz)	64±11	28	179
RASPBERRY, 100% fruit spread, 25g (0.9oz)	26±4	3	42
RAVIOLI, meat-filled, 180g (6.3oz)	39±1	15	344
RICE, Basmati white, 150g (5.3oz)	57±4	22	268
RICE, brown, cooked, 150g (5.3oz)	50	16	165
RICE, instant, white, cooked, 150g (5.3oz)	74±10	31	174
RICE, sticky, cooked, 150g (5.3oz)	87±2	24	146
RICE, Uncle Ben's Ready Whole Grain, Brown, 140g (4.4oz)	48	20	190
RICE, white, cooked, 150g (5.3oz)	72±8	29	194
RICE CAKES, puffed caramel flavored, 25g (0.9oz)	82±10	18	95
RICE CAKES, puffed plain, 25g (0.9oz)	82±11	17	97
SLIM FAST, chocolate meal replacement bar, 50g (1.8oz)	27±3	6	200
SLIM FAST, vanilla shake, 250mL (1.1cup)	37±5	10	153
SOFT DRINK, Coca Cola, 250mL (1.1cup)	63	16	102

Fat (grams)	Carbs (grams)	Fiber (grams)	Sugar (grams)	Protein (grams)
5	25	1	2	4
8	16	1	2	3
5	24	2	2	3
19	25	2	2	3
1	24	1	1	3
0	47	3	45	2
0	38	5	26	2
3	19	1	12	3
3	19	0	17	3
0	5	0	1	1
7	27	3	4	33
10	27	2	3	32
3	40	3	0	8
0	48	2	36	2
0	10	0	10	0
13	31	1	1	23
2	57	1	0	5
1	34	3	1	4
1	37	1	0	3
0	32	2	0	3
3	39	3	0	5
0	42	1	0	4
0	21	0	6	2
1	20	1	0	2
6	25	1	23	10
5	20	4	15	9
0	28	0	28	0

Description of food	Glycemic index	Glycemic load (per serving)	Calories (kcal)
SOFT DRINK, Fanta orange, 250mL (1.1cup)	68	23	160
SOUP, minestrone, Campbell's, 250g (8.8oz)	48±6	18	114
SOUP, tomato, Campbell's, 250g (8.8oz)	52±4	15	187
SOY MILK, whole, 250mL (1.1cup)	44±5	8	135
SPLIT PEAS, yellow, boiled, 150g (5.3oz)	25±6	3	177
STRAWBERRIES, fresh, 120g (4.2oz)	40±7	1	38
STRAWBERRY, fruit leather, 30g (1.1oz)	29±4	7	90
STRAWBERRY, 100% fruit spread, 30g (1.1oz)	46±5	8	58
STRAWBERRY JAM, 30g (1.1oz)	51±10	10	75
STUFFED GRAPEVINE LEAVES (rice, lamb, & tomato), 100g (3.5oz)	30±11	5	266
SWEET POTATO, 150g (5.3oz)	70±6	22	129
TOMATO JUICE, 250mL (1.1cup)	31	2	44
TORTILLA, corn, 50g (1.8oz)	52	12	109
TORTILLA, wheat, 50g (1.8oz)	30	8	132
VEGETABLE JUICE, V8, 250mL (1.1cup)	43±4	4	52
VEGGIE BURGER, vegetable patty with bun, 100g (3.5oz)	59±8	14	177
WATERMELON, fresh, 120g (4.2oz)	72±13	4	36
YAM, 150g (5.3oz)	54±8	20	177
YOGURT, low fat, flavored, with sugar, 200g (7.1oz)	33±3	11	170
YOGURT, low fat, fruit, artificially sweetened, 200g (7.1oz)	14±4	2	210
YOGURT, low fat, fruit, with sugar, 200g (7.1oz)	33±7	10	204
YOGURT, plain, 200g (7.1oz)	19±6	3	126
YOGURT, Yoplait, no fat, artificially sweetened, flavored, 200g (7.1oz)	18±1	2	105

Fat (grams)	Carbs (grams)	Fiber (grams)	Sugar (grams)	Protein (grams)
0	45	0	44	0
1	21	3	7	5
0	42	2	25	4
5	13	3	1	12
1	32	13	4	13
0	9	2	6	1
0	24	2	18	0
0	15	0	15	0
0	20	0	18	0
21	12	3	2	8
0	30	5	6	2
0	11	1	9	2
1	22	3	1	3
1	28	4	2	5
0	10	2	8	2
6	14	5	1	16
0	9	1	7	1
0	42	6	1	2
3	28	0	28	10
3	37	0	6	10
2	38	0	38	9
3	14	0	14	11
0	19	0	12	6

NOTES: